PARAMEDICS ON AND OFF THE STREETS

Emergency Medical Services in the Age of Technological Governance

In *Paramedics On and Off the Streets*, Michael K. Corman embarks on an institutional ethnography of the complex, mundane, intricate, and exhilarating work of paramedics in Calgary, Alberta.

Corman's comprehensive research includes more than 200 hours of participant observation ride-alongs with paramedics over a period of eleven months, more than 100 interviews with paramedics, and thirty-six interviews with other emergency medical personnel including administrators, call-takers and dispatchers, nurses, and doctors. At the heart of this ethnography are questions about the role of paramedics in urban environments, the role of information and communication technologies in contemporary health care governance, and the organization and accountability of pre-hospital medical services. *Paramedics On and Off the Streets* is the first institutional ethnography to explore the role and increasing importance of paramedics in our healthcare system. It takes readers on a journey into the everyday lives of EMS personnel and provides an in-depth sociological analysis of the work of pre-hospital health care professionals in the twenty-first century.

MICHAEL K. CORMAN is a principal advisor in the Department of Health and Wellness for the Government of Prince Edward Island and an adjunct professor in the Department of Sociology & Anthropology and Faculty of Nursing at the University of Prince Edward Island, Canada.

T0260651

Paramedics On and Off the Streets

Emergency Medical Services in the Age of Technological Governance

MICHAEL K. CORMAN

UNIVERSITY OF TORONTO PRESS
Toronto Buffalo London

© University of Toronto Press 2017
Toronto Buffalo London
www.utppublishing.com

ISBN 978-1-4426-2986-8 (cloth)
ISBN 978-1-4426-2987-5 (paper)

Library and Archives Canada Cataloguing in Publication

Corman, Michael K., 1982–, author
Paramedics on and off the streets : emergency medical services in the age of
technological governance / Michael K. Corman.

Includes bibliographical references and index.
ISBN 978-1-4426-2986-8 (cloth). – ISBN 978-1-4426-2987-5 (paper)

1. Emergency medical services – Alberta – Calgary.   2. Allied health
personnel – Alberta – Calgary.   I. Title.

RA996.C32C35 2017   362.18097123'38   C2017-902551-1

This book has been published with the help of a grant from the Federation
for the Humanities and Social Sciences, through the Awards to Scholarly
Publications Program, using funds provided by the Social Sciences and
Humanities Research Council of Canada.

University of Toronto Press acknowledges the financial assistance to its
publishing program of the Canada Council for the Arts and the Ontario
Arts Council, an agency of the Government of Ontario.

Canada Council   Conseil des Arts
for the Arts   du Canada

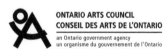

ONTARIO ARTS COUNCIL
CONSEIL DES ARTS DE L'ONTARIO

an Ontario government agency
un organisme du gouvernement de l'Ontario

Funded by the   Financé par le
Government   gouvernement
of Canada   du Canada

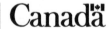

Canadä

*To Harvey and Gabe, forever you will be in
my heart and I in yours*

Contents

List of Figures

Acknowledgments

This research would not have been possible without all of the people who agreed to participate. Thank you for welcoming me into your work settings and allowing me to talk to you and observe you *at work*. And especially to all of the paramedics with whom I spent so much time at all hours of day in so many different contexts, thank you for taking the time to "teach me as if I were to do your work." I hope this book explicates the complexities of what you do. I also had support from Alberta Health Services, Emergency Medical Services, and financial support through the Social Science and Humanities Research Council of Canada, to do this research, without which it would not have been possible.

This book is the culmination of nearly 10 years of research and writing. Over the years, I have had significant support from many people, specifically Kiara Okita, Aime McLean, Carol Berenson, Jason Hickey, Sita Fox, Shannon Blanke, and Kim Critchley. Early on in this research, I was invited by Dorothy Smith and Alison Griffith to participate in a workshop on governance in society at York University. This workshop allowed me to discuss and think about my research in a setting that was informative and insightful. After the workshop, I developed a working relationship and friendship with Karen Melon, with whom I worked on a publication. Our collaboration was informative and contributed to my thinking of the pre-hospital and emergency department interface. Similarly, my participation in the Institutional Ethnography division of the Society for the Study of Social Problems over the years also allowed me to think about my research in an environment with other institutional ethnographers that facilitated my process of discovery.

Throughout phases of this research, I have received critical feedback from Arthur Frank, Janet Rankin, Lauren Eastwood, and Ariel Ducey, all of whom are exemplary scholars. Furthermore, I was fortunate to work with Janet at the University of Calgary in Qatar, where we had many "problematic" conversations about my research and institutional ethnography, all of which informed my thinking. Janet's book with Marie Campbell, *Managing to Nurse: Inside Canada's Health Care Reform*, along with Timothy Diamond's book, *Making Gray Gold: Narratives of Nursing Home Care*, were seminal in my thinking and writing of this book. Also, thank you to Marjorie DeVault and Eric Mykhalovskiy for providing a thorough and critical review of the book and offering suggestions to improve this manuscript, and to Stephen Shapiro and Lisa Jemison, my editors at the University of Toronto Press, whose knowledge of the publication process and timely and pragmatic feedback greatly aided me in getting this to print.

I have been lucky to have had outstanding mentors throughout my years in the academy. I remember very clearly my first institutional ethnography seminar, which I took from Dorothy Smith at the University of Victoria. This class, and the unwavering mentorship and support from Dorothy that followed, set the foundation for my scholarship and desire to explore "how things work" in different institutional settings. Liza McCoy, my mentor, colleague, and friend, supported me throughout this research; without her continuous guidance, wisdom, and, most of all, patience, this research would not have been realized.

Lastly, to Glenda and Doug, you have been with me on this journey from the beginning to the end, listening to me, putting up with me, and caring for me. To my father, your passion for what you do has invariably contributed to my passion for what I do. And, of course, to *My One and Only* – Tara – thank you for your continued support, editorial prowess, and unconditional partnership.

Permissions

Some of the material in this book also appears in my article entitled "Street Medicine: Assessment Work Strategies of Paramedics on the Front Lines of Emergency Health Services," published in the *Journal of Contemporary Ethnography* in 2016.

List of Abbreviations

AAIMS	Alberta Ambulance Information Management System
AH	Alberta Health
AHS	Alberta Health Services
AHW	Alberta Health and Wellness
ALS	Advanced Life Support
BLS	Basic Life Support
CA	conversational analysis
CAD	Computer Aided Dispatch
CHAPS	Community Health and Pre-hospital Support
CIHI	Canadian Institute for Health Information
DAD	Discharge Abstract Database
EBM	evidence-based medicine
ED	emergency department
EMD	Emergency Medical Dispatch
EMR	Emergency Medical Responder
EMS	Emergency Medical Services
EMT	Emergency Medical Technician
EMT-P	Emergency Medical Technologist-Paramedic
ePCR	Electronic Patient Care Record/Report
HQCA	Health Quality Council of Alberta
ICTs	information and communication technologies
IE	institutional ethnography
NACRS	National Ambulatory Care Reporting System
OECD	Organisation for Economic Cooperation and Development
PCR	patient care record/report
REDIS	Regional Emergency Department Information Systems
REPAC	Regional Emergency Patient Access and Coordination system

SAIT   Southern Alberta Institute of Technology
SOPs   standard operating procedures
SSM   system status management
WHO   World Health Organization

PARAMEDICS ON AND OFF THE STREETS

Emergency Medical Services in the
Age of Technological Governance

Chapter One

Introduction

Opening Vignette ... Getting Hooked

Most people at some point in their life will come face-to-face with paramedics. This was the case for me in 2009 while driving my partner to work. In the act of turning into a parking lot, our car collided with an individual riding a bicycle. I remember glass everywhere, levels of adrenaline never experienced, and a loud scream. I called 911 to report the accident and request an ambulance to assist the cyclist, who sat in pain on the curb, bleeding, sweating, and in tears. The call-taker asked certain questions, along the lines of "Are you in need of police, fire, or ambulance?" and "Is the individual conscious?" Time passed and the paramedics eventually arrived. One paramedic immediately approached the cyclist, asked her some questions, and then appeared to examine different body parts. Another paramedic approached my partner and me. A brief encounter followed, no body checks, only questions asked. Moments later, the paramedic turned away and assisted the other paramedic in loading the injured cyclist onto a stretcher and eventually into the ambulance. Soon, the ambulance left, off to what I could only presume was a hospital, lights glaring, sirens blaring.

As I reflected on this experience, I contrasted my observations with my own conceptions of emergency medical services (EMS) and the work of paramedics. One image of EMS work that I had was of paramedics as passive health care workers who simply drove patients to the hospital with minimal involvement in patient care. Contradicting this was another image I had of paramedics as heroic lifesavers who provided medical intervention to those experiencing a medical crisis. These stereotypical images likely derived from popular portrayals of paramedics represented in different forms of media I had been exposed to.

My interests in EMS and the work of paramedics[1] was activated by this experience. I became intrigued and puzzled by the interactions between the paramedics and me, my partner, and the cyclist, and what happened once the paramedics left with the cyclist. I began to wonder about the work of paramedics – what do they do? – and how their work is organized at the accident site and beyond. Suffice it to say, I was hooked and wanted to learn more about EMS broadly and the work of paramedics specifically. I wanted to learn more about how things work in EMS from the standpoint of paramedics.

Being a "Good" Academic

Historical Roots of EMS and Paramedics

Having my interest piqued, and as a "good" academic, I delved into the literature on EMS and paramedics. I learned that the historical roots of emergency service workers and "the ambulance" likely began in ancient Greece and grew out of an attempt to transport, and eventually treat, soldiers who were wounded in battle (see Bell, 2009; Chung, 2001). The history of EMS in Canada began in the 1800s when the St John's Ambulance opened its first Canadian Branch in Quebec to teach individuals first aid (Health Quality Council of Alberta [HQCA], 2013).[2] Prior to the 1970s, ambulance service "attendants" or "drivers" in North America lacked medical training and equipment and were primarily tasked with getting their patient(s) to the closest hospital as quickly as possible – "you call, we haul" – with limited, if any, medical intervention (Bergman, 2007; Palmer, 1989). Much of this pre-hospital care was even done by morticians, with an obvious conflict of interest (Metz, 1981). Furthermore, services were minimally regulated, if at all (Metz, 1981; Shah, 2006). Critics during this time suggested that the procedures used were outdated and lacked regulation and minimum standards, and thus reforming them should "be given the highest priority in our efforts to improve the nation's health" (Metz, 1981, p. 4).

Contemporary EMS in North America can be traced back to the 1960s with the passage of National Acts (Suter, 2012) and subsequent standards, policies, and practices that began to regulate the work of pre-hospital emergency care personnel at the federal level in the United States (Shah, 2006) and at the provincial level in Canada (HQCA, 2013).

These developments essentially created "a new health professional" known as the emergency medical technician (EMT) (Metz, 1981, p. 5). Following these developments was the establishment of EMS in different regions throughout North America and the development of emergency dispatching systems that allowed for the activation and coordination of pre-hospital emergency medical services (Metz, 1981). These institutional changes to the context of EMS, along with the institutionalization of emergency medicine as a sub-specialty in medicine and nursing (Metz, 1981, Suter, 2012), brought significant advances in the training of, and level of care administered by, paramedics in the United States and Canada.

In Alberta, legislative Acts cemented the role of EMS in the province from the 1980s onwards. The Health Disciplines Act,[3] for example, was amended in the mid-1980s to include paramedics as health care practitioners who, under the oversight of a physician, known as "medical control," could perform a variety of interventions depending on their level of training (discussed below) (HQCA, 2013). Furthermore, the Emergency Health Services Act of 2008, which replaced the Ambulance Services Act of 1994, gave responsibility to the province to set regulations for ambulance vehicles, EMS workers, and dispatch services in the province (HQCA, 2013). Suffice it to say, over the last 40 years, pre-hospital emergency medical services have transitioned from what may be thought of as a group of ancillary workers with little training and education to an occupational group and organizational site integral to "the provision of health care" (Alberta Health and Wellness [AHW], 2008a, p. 12). The paramedic's unique skill-set and ability to function in diverse situations have resulted in the occupation becoming ever more important to health care systems (AHW, 2008a, p. 12). Paramedics now make up a significant portion of health care workers in Canada and the United States, with numbers exceeding 30,000 and over a quarter of a million respectively in each country (Bureau of Labor Statistics, 2015; Paramedics Association of Canada, 2011).

As paramedics become increasingly integrated into the health care system, their work necessarily interfaces with that of other front-line workers, including doctors, nurses, and other health practitioners in hospital settings. However, research in the sociological study of health and health care that explores the work of health care professionals focuses primarily on doctors and nurses, which gives the false impression, as Ducey (2009) notes, that "physicians and registered nurses are the only care providers at the bedside" (p. 3). Combine this with the fact

that paramedics and emergency medical services are undergoing significant changes (discussed below), and it is clear that the profession and
the work setting of paramedics are ripe for sociological investigation.

Paramedics' Training and Organizational Oversight

Paramedics are trained to use specialized medical knowledge and
a variety of medical procedures and pharmaceutical interventions
to "save patients and prevent further damage" in emergency situations, both as members of "health-care teams" in hospital emergency
departments (Swanson, 2005, p. 96) and *on the streets* – unpredictable
environments "rife with chaotic, dangerous, and often uncontrollable
elements" (Nelson, 1997, cited in Campeau, 2008, p. 3). In Canada, the
paramedic profession generally consists of three designations of pre-
hospital emergency care workers: the Emergency Medical Responder
(EMR), the Emergency Medical Technician (EMT), and the Emergency
Medical Technologist-Paramedic (EMT-P). Each designation is differen-
tiated by the amount of training and education, in-the-field experience,
and scope of practice.

In Calgary, Alberta, where my research was conducted, the Southern Alberta Institute of Technology (SAIT)[4] offers a 176-hour EMR program where individuals learn about emergency medical services, how
ambulances operate, and pertinent skills, such as "patient assessment,
basic life support, trauma and medical emergencies, pediatrics, child-
birth, geriatrics, environmental, psychological and special situations."
Once a person has achieved EMR designation by passing a provincial
examination, they are eligible for EMT certification. SAIT also offers a
10-month EMT certificate program. This program "covers all aspects of
prehospital emergency care, including Advanced Life Support, patient
assessment, diagnostics, treatment and critical interventions." Classes
include anatomy and physiology, patient assessment, basic pharmacology, traumatic emergencies, respiratory emergencies, health and safety,
professional practice, medical terminology, medical emergencies,
special populations, cardiac emergencies, and two practica in order
to "apply theory and skills learned under the direct supervision of a
preceptor."

Finally, in order to train EMT-Ps, SAIT offers a full-time, two-year
program to EMTs. This program allows students to "become exten-
sively familiar with human anatomy, physiology and pathophysiology,
as well as a wide variety of pharmacological and other therapies."

In addition, classes attempt to facilitate the development of critical thinking skills and train individuals to use different advanced procedures and skills, such as fluid resuscitation and rapid sequence induction. The curriculum also includes different practica, including clinical rotations in hospital emergency and operation rooms. Both EMTs and EMT-Ps have to pass a provincial examination in order to work in the province.

Overseeing the training of paramedics is the regulatory body that governs paramedics. In Alberta, this body is known as the Alberta College of Paramedics. The College determines paramedics' scope of practice – what paramedics can and cannot do – based on their designation (e.g., EMR, EMT, EMT-P), sets standards for education programs in the province, and is responsible for registering and renewing registration of paramedics. In order for paramedics to practise in the province, they must be registered with the College. It is important to note that while the College legally determines scope of practice, paramedics work under the licence of physicians known as medical directors. As such, while the scope of practice outlines what paramedics can and cannot do at the level of their professional designation, medical directors determine standard operating procedures or protocols that determine what paramedics can and cannot do to their patients depending on the jurisdiction in which they work.

Key changes to the organizational oversight occurred for paramedics in Alberta in 2009 when the provincial government took over EMS, including the service in Calgary. Prior to this reform, the City of Calgary was responsible for running pre-hospital emergency services. While major reforms implemented in 2009 played out during this research, it is important to view these changes as a process connected to past reforms that date back to 1993 or earlier. In 1993, Alberta implemented the regionalization of health care services, "motivated by financial and quality goals. Provincial leaders believed that regional governance could generate cost savings and improved health care services through economies of scale and coordination of services" (Baker et al., 2008, p. 221). As a result, "over 100 hospital boards and 27 public health unit boards were abolished" in order to create 17 regional health authorities, "each under a single board and budget" (Wilson, 2007, p. 167). The regional authorities were "responsible for the planning and delivery of hospital-based, continuing, community-based and public healthcare services" (Baker et al., 2008, p. 221). These 17 authorities were later consolidated to nine regional authorities in 2003.

The 2009 reform consolidated these health authorities under one provincial health authority, known as Alberta Health Services (AHS), with the overarching mantra, "We Are One – One team. One Board. One plan for the delivery of health care in Alberta."[5] Similar to past justifications for health care restructuring, this reform was implemented "to enhance health care and develop an approach that places the patient first regardless of where they live in Alberta."[6] According to governmental bodies in Alberta, centralization "has created a unique opportunity to reinvent the health services operating model and to increase the effectiveness of Alberta's health care system" (AHW, 2008a, p. 3), essentially "mak[ing] the province's system more efficient and effective."[7]

Furthermore, and connecting to new managerialism (discussed below), one of the major goals of this reform is to better manage and coordinate health services and health service workers in the province. As AHW (2008a) explains:

> To meet [today's health care] challenges, Alberta Health and Wellness can facilitate decisions that promote access, quality, and sustainability. This will require (1) actively managing the factors that can reduce demand for the costliest and least-efficient health care services; (2) ensuring that health care supply matches the quality, timeliness, and cost-effectiveness that Albertans require; and (3) creating a delivery mechanism that facilitates equilibrium between supply and demand. (p. 5)

Classifying, generalizing, and standardizing were central tenets to the 2009 reform and the achievement of this goal. AHW (2008a), for instance, suggests that a "significant variation exists in the way care is delivered in institutions across Alberta" (p. 39); therefore, this reform seeks to standardize care across the province to increase and enhance quality of care and increase system efficiency by "standardiz[ing] data collection, and collaborat[ing] to expand best practices across Alberta" (p. 44).

Paramedics' Work

Through my review of the literature, I learned that it had been a long time since the work of EMS had garnered serious sociological attention. During the early 1970s and 1980s, for example, a few sociologists were drawn to study paramedics because the occupation, as well as emergency medical services more generally, was a relatively new profession and was under transition. This research contributed to a better understanding of what paramedics do by providing a variety of accounts that depicted the diversity of calls and patients paramedics encountered. Such research also shed light on the culture of paramedics; job-related stressors; the structure of the organization the paramedics were embedded within; and the interaction between paramedics and other individuals, including emergency (police and fire) and medical personnel, the patients' families, bystanders, and media personnel (Metz, 1981, Palmer, 1983a; 1983b; 1989).

This research also discussed the different types of roles paramedics play. For example, there is the role of the "medical authority figure," whereby the patient(s), bystanders, and law enforcement and fire department personnel rely on the work of paramedics to "take over" the scene of accidents and "restore the status quo to the street" (Palmer, 1983a, pp. 173–4). When this role, and the respect that goes along with it, is not achieved, Palmer suggests that this can lead to "role strain." Other roles include that of "lifesaver," "information specialist" (collecting important administrative and patient information), the "partner" role with other paramedics, and the role of fulfilling "other work duties," such as ensuring that needed medical supplies are in the ambulance and the ambulance unit is clean.

In addition to focusing on the different roles of paramedics, Palmer described paramedics as "trauma junkies," who get, and come to need, a psychological "high," depending on the type of call, or "run," as it is known colloquially. In other words, paramedics become "hooked" on the work of practising pre-hospital emergency care. The "high," Palmer argues, is dependent on the perceived quality of the call, with "good" calls requiring advanced medical intervention; such calls are "exciting, quick paced, action packed, [and] successful" (Palmer, 1983a, p. 164). This is in contrast to "shit" runs; calls that are viewed as "nonessential," such as domestic abuse and "nonemergency calls" (Palmer, 1983a, p. 167). Palmer further argues that "good" runs are essential for the well-being of paramedics, resulting in paramedics having a positive image of themselves and reduced mental health problems (e.g., depression and anxiety).

In more recent sociological research, Nurok and Henckes (2009) explore how the different professional values of emergency service workers[8] compete with each other and impact the care provided to patients. For example, the value of patients based on social categories of "age, sex, race, and socio-economic status can be inferred" by the paramedic (p. 506) and potentially mediates the care the emergency worker provides. These researchers also draw attention to how the difficulty of a call, the level of trauma a patient is experiencing, and the chance of "saving" a patient can compete with how paramedics orient to the "social value" of patients; the patients that emergency workers treat are valued differently, and these values conflict or align at times depending on the context of the call.

Other research has examined EMS work from a psychosocial perspective or has been concerned more with "operational" issues in emergency services. Psychosocial research has investigated coping strategies and resources paramedics use to deal with the demands of their work, recruitment and retention issues, and job-related stress (see, for example, Donnelly, 2012). Operational research has been concerned with the accuracy of emergency medical dispatchers in classifying the severity of calls (Clawson, Olola, Heward, Scott, & Patterson, 2007), what individual qualities are "desirable" for being a paramedic (Kilner, 2004a; b), and the training of paramedics (Boyle, Williams, & Burgess, 2007) and their experiences with training (Boyle, Williams, Cooper, Adams, & Alford, 2008).

Why Paramedics? Why Now?

EMS and the work of paramedics connect inevitably to contemporary notions of "modern" healthcare and understandings of life and death; whether you realize it or not, paramedics are an occupational group that you will likely come into contact with at some point in your life in an unplanned manner. EMS and the work of paramedics exist in every major city and in many rural areas throughout North America and other countries around the world (Emergency Medical Services Chiefs of Canada, 2006; see also Roudsari et al., 2007). In North America, EMS treat and/or transport approximately 2 million individuals in Canada and between 25 and 30 million individuals in the United States annually (Emergency Medical Services Chiefs of Canada, 2006; National EMS Research Agenda, 2001). In Alberta alone, a province with over 3 million people, pre-hospital emergency medical services respond to nearly 400,000 "ambulance events" annually (Alberta Health Services [AHS], 2011).

Furthermore, according to the Canadian Institute for Health Information (2005), roughly 12 per cent of those visiting the emergency department arrive by ambulance. However, of those who visit the emergency department with "the most severe health concerns" (p. 6), 78 per cent are transported by an ambulance. Similar numbers exist in the United States, with 16 million of 114 million visits to an emergency department arriving by an ambulance (Institute of Medicine (US), 2007). EMS has also been described as the "safety net of the safety net" because in addition to providing care to those in emergent and traumatic situations, it also provides care to those with limited or no access to health and social services (p. xv). Hence, the work of paramedics transgresses social and economic boundaries, treating and/or transporting individuals ranging from those with higher social and economic status to vulnerable persons, such as individuals who are homeless, substance users, those who have mental health issues and/or developmental disabilities, and other individuals at risk of abuse, neglect, social exclusion, and economic hardships. Lastly, as Al-Shaqsi (2010) notes, EMS is often "the first point of contact for the majority of people to health care services during emergencies and life-threatening injuries and act[s] as a gate-keeping step for accessing secondary and tertiary services" (p. 320).

As discussed, the early research on paramedics' work provides descriptions of the work paramedics do and primarily took place following the institutionalization of pre-hospital emergency care in the 1970s. However, much has changed, and continues to change, since the early years of emergency health services. In addition to advances in paramedics' training, there have been many advances in the field of emergency medicine in terms of treatments, both surgical and pharmacological, which have translated into increased levels of medical intervention that paramedics can now do on the streets. In other words, the type and number of interventions paramedics have available today is vastly different from what was available to them in the earlier years of the profession. Concomitant with increased medical interventions are advances in medical technologies, which now allow paramedics to perform a variety of diagnostic procedures and medical interventions that historically were not possible (e.g., electrocardiograms (ECGs), oxygen, and blood sugar level readings).

Also of significance to contemporary EMS, and to health care more generally, are advances in information and communication technologies (ICTs) that allow for the tracking and coordination of EMS and paramedics, not to mention a better ability to communicate with other EMS personnel while on and off the streets. In other words, differing from the past, when Metz (1981) explains that paramedics were "free from close supervision" (p. 66) and the "Company does not have any routine measures for checking the quality of patient care, nor does the city, nor the state" (p. 187), new technologies have been introduced to govern the work of those on the front line of pre-hospital care. Some specific examples of such technologies in Calgary include the Regional Emergency Patient Access and Coordination system (REPAC), which is a technology used to coordinate EMS; computer-assisted devices located in ambulances; global positioning systems; and electronic patient care records used by paramedics. All of these technologies connect to different information collection and tracking systems in the province and evidence-based protocols that structure what paramedics can and cannot do. These technologies are central to what gets counted as "quality of care."

The lack of research on the work and workplace settings of contemporary urban paramedics is particularly worrisome in light of how paramedics and their work settings are being targeted by health care reform and restructuring practices geared towards solving different crises that have plagued contemporary health care systems (Goldman, 2008). Such crises include overcrowding and increased wait times for patients in emergency department settings, increased costs of health care, concerns over the quality of care that patients receive in emergency settings, and lack of accountability in the health arena.[9] All of the ICTs discussed above are in one way or another geared towards addressing such crises and therefore connect to reform and restructuring practices in Canada.

Integral to these reform practices in health care, and central to the workplace setting of contemporary paramedics, are *new forms and technologies of knowledge and governance* – "forms of language, technologies of representation and communication, and text-based, objectified modes of knowledge through which local particularities are interpreted or rendered actionable in abstract, translocal terms" (McCoy, 2008, p. 701). Central to this age of technological governance in health care are ideologies of *neoliberalism* and *new managerialism* or *new public management* (Rankin & Campbell, 2006; Armstrong, Armstrong, & Scott-Dixon, 2008; Williams et al., 2001). Neoliberalism refers to the idea that successful private sector market-based solutions are most apt to solve public sector problems – abstract market processes are conceived as being the best way to organize human life (DeVault, 2008).

Related to neoliberalism, and integral to its implementation in practice, is the ethos of new managerialism or new public management. This ethos attempts to promote the market ideals of efficiency and accountability through the management of people's work by and through new forms and technologies of knowledge and governance (DeVault, 2008, pp. 12–13).[10] Through "optimal" coordination and close monitoring of services, for example, it is believed that the "flow" of patients through the system can be better managed, therefore leading to increased efficiencies (AHW, 2008a, p. 38). Accordingly, principles of new managerialism are being proposed with the goal of garnering system efficiencies by applying "operations management principles to help streamline care and remove waste" (p. 41). This is especially relevant for EMS, as they are being targeted by reforms aimed at expanding their role in the province and making their work more efficient through monitoring and coordination.

Together, these discourses, and the restructuring practices in the public sector that are organized by them, have become pervasive throughout many if not all sectors of society (Clarke & Newman, 1997; Daniel, 2008); they are central to contemporary health care reforms in Alberta, which has historically preferred neoliberal styles of management and governance (Church & Smith, 2006), and in Canada. However, such reforms are not unique to Canada or the health care industry (Barnett et al., 1998; Brown, 2006; Cochrane, 2004; Cribb, 2008; Hall, 2005); neoliberalism and new managerialism have become a hegemonic hybrid (Cribb, 2008) pervasive throughout society, and concomitant to the *managerial state* (Clarke & Newman, 1997; Daniel, 2008). As Clarke and Newman (1997) explain, "it is difficult to find any reform in the last decade which has not drawn on and contributed to the installation of a managerial mode of coordination – from the creation of Civil Service Agencies to the reorganisation of health and social care around market relations" (p. 60).

Implemented by health practitioners and policy makers alike, these ideologically organized forms and technologies of knowledge and governance have become a "paradigm" for the health arena, organizing and coordinating health care policy and practice with the goal of fine-tuning health systems and health workers in order to make them more efficient, effective, and transparent, all while improving patient care (Mykhalovskiy & Weir, 2004, p. 1060; Rankin & Campbell, 2006). They attempt to do so by intervening into how practitioners do their work and how their work is made accountable. New forms and technologies of knowledge and governance are essential for the organization, coordination, and objectification of work on the front line; they are essential for making health practitioners' work accountable to management and government by filtering local happenings through regulatory discourses embedded within textual technologies for purposes of measuring, monitoring, and managing medical work and health care (Hogle, 2008; Wholey & Burns, 2000). In Alberta (and elsewhere), governance, defined here as inter-institutional ways of organizing and coordinating people's doings through translocal text-mediated and text-regulated relations activated by people (see DeVault, 2008, pp. 9–13),[11] is at the nexus of health care, health practice, and health relations, facilitated by technological and bureaucratic complexes (Zola, 1972, p. 487). Although governance is central to the work of contemporary paramedics, it has failed to garner serious sociological attention.

Essentially, change is afoot in what paramedics do and how their work is being organized and reorganized in the age of technological governance. From a social scientific perspective, there is very little known about the work of paramedics in the 21st century, making the occupation "rich with unexplored opportunities for research on the full range of paramedic work" (Campeau, 2008, p. 2). It is especially important to understand how the work of paramedics is changing in light of recent health care reforms because 1) Reforms are often characterized by dilemmas and hardships for those living through them, since they are often ambiguous in nature and characterized by uncertain developments (Clarke & Newman, 1997, p. 50); and 2) Those on the front line often bear the brunt of reforms – "frontline health care workers are always most vulnerable to the perpetual tides of health care 'reform'" – having to carry out and adjust their work to a changing social organization in which their work is embedded (Ducey, 2009, p. 6). Furthermore, it is these front-line workers who "are the most insightful critics of what is wrong with how health care work is organized and care delivered" (p. 14).

Exploring how the work of paramedics is organized and interfaces with the work of other health care professionals, administrators, and a multiplicity of managerial technologies will allow for a better understanding of how things work in the emergency medical complex. In doing so, this book answers to Rankin and Campbell's (2006) call for additional research that explores how knowledge in health care is put together in ways that "may accomplish its ruling purposes but otherwise fail people and, moreover, obscure that failure" (p. 182). Furthermore, this empirical investigation draws attention to the benefits and "hidden dangers" (Rankin & Campbell, 2006; Campbell, 2008) of new forms and technologies of knowledge and governance that are central to the ongoing changes to the emergency medical complex and the broader health care system. What we learn is that rather than the patient and practitioner being centre-stage in the governance of health care on the front lines of EMS, narrow conceptions of efficiency and accountability are infiltrating the work settings of paramedics and displacing both patients and practitioners as knowing subjects, with problematic and unforeseen consequences. Exploring the work of paramedics in relation to how reform and restructuring practices are "accomplished on the ground" (DeVault, 2008, p. 9) makes meaningful change more likely. This book, then, is situated at the intersection of the work of paramedics and the significant changes to how pre-hospital emergency health care services are organized and coordinated in the 21st century.

Purpose of the Book

This book explores the work of paramedics in the context of significant changes in EMS. More specifically, I explore what paramedics do – their work processes – and I explicate how the work of urban paramedics is socially organized in contemporary society by different *institutional technologies*: "the specific tools that workers use to accomplish their tasks and the institutionally organized procedures for accomplishing these tasks" (Pence 2001, p. 204). This book, therefore, speaks to three interrelated questions or "puzzles" that were activated by my encounter with paramedics discussed at the outset of this chapter:

1) What do urban paramedics actually do on the front lines of pre-hospital emergency medical services?
2) How does the work of paramedics interface with other workers in EMS?
3) How is the work of paramedics organized, coordinated, and made institutionally accountable?

By exploring these three interrelated questions, this book first and foremost provides readers with a vibrant account of key players in EMS and describes what paramedics do as they interface with their patients; my detailed description of paramedics' ordinary and extraordinary work is nuanced and complex.[12] In addition, I show how the work of paramedics is being structured as though it is ordinary and simple. I ethnographically look beyond the promise of technological innovation and explore how technological changes play out in practice, often with hidden consequences. In doing so, the analytical contribution of this book is 1) to provide a socio-historical context of pre-hospital emergency services work, 2) to investigate how paramedics' work is being organized and restructured with "accounting logics" (Diamond, 1992) and discourses of neoliberalism and new managerialism mediated by technological "innovations," and 3) to explore, as Ducey (2009) notes, "who gains – and who does not" from current reform and "reengineering" practices that target the work of those on the front line (p. 5). This book also provides individuals interested in how health care is being reformed and restructured in the age of technological governance with important evidence to reflect upon in terms of how things do and do not work. Such an analysis is not only relevant to neoliberal reform and restructuring practices in health care but also points to broader changes happening in the public sector and their consequences.

In and Out of the Field

To explore the work of paramedics and how their work is organized, the research upon which this book is based was designed as an institutional ethnography (IE) (Smith, 2005, 1987). This design facilitated the exploration of the complex interface between "'what actually happens'" (Campbell & Gregor, 2002, p. 52) *on the streets* of pre-hospital emergency medical services and how those happenings are institutionally organized and put together *off the streets*. I began by observing paramedics "on the street" and in the hospital in order to ethnographically observe the day-to-day vicissitudes on the front line and learn about the reality of paramedics' work (Diamond, 1992, p. 247 n. 8) and the technologies they use, and to see first hand the kinds of situations that arise. Observations occurred during the normal work hours of paramedics. During observation shifts, I rode along with paramedics in the back of the ambulance, typically in the airway seat (see chapter 2), though where I sat during a ride-along depended on whether a student was also with the crew and the preferences of the crew, which sometimes changed according to the needs of the patient. These ride-alongs occurred during a period of 11 months between December 2010 and October 2011.[13] Over these 11 months, I observed paramedics for a total of 212.75 hours during 34 separate ride-alongs. I rode with 14 unique paramedic pairs[14] and observed 24 paramedics in total.

As a participant observer, I was a "known observer." This meant that the paramedics were fully aware that there was a researcher doing a study (Mannon, 1982). While observing, I took a "participating-to-write" approach to writing my fieldnotes (Emerson et al., 2011, p. 23).[15] I informed participants that I would be taking extensive "jottings" (notes) with the goal of producing "a more detailed, closer-to-the-moment record" of what paramedics do (p. 22). My goal was to establish a "note-taker" role very early on during my observations so that it became commonplace for my participants to see me writing extensive jottings. The jottings included keywords and phrases about what I had observed, and sometimes included verbatim talk from participants. I used a small notebook that fitted in my back pocket. If it was inappropriate to jot notes in the field (e.g., in the midst of a medical crisis or when family members were present), then I took notes when a more appropriate time emerged (once the patient was transferred to hospital, during a break, en route to hospital, etc.). My jottings focused on the work involved with being a paramedic and how this work is hooked up with the institutional complex in which it occurs.

My initial jottings were expanded into full fieldnotes immediately following observations. I did this in order to retain the nuances of what would inevitably become more commonplace the longer I was in the field. The writing of these initial fieldnotes sometimes took three to four days, as I found writing extensive fieldnotes based on a six-, eight-, or twelve-hour shift took much time. As I spent more time in the field, I still took extensive jottings, but only expanded on jottings of observations that I found "interesting." Some of these "interesting" events shocked or angered me; such events "may also reflect contradictory pressures experienced by those in the setting" (Emerson et al., 2011, p. 25). Other observations focused on similarities and/or differences in relation to previous observations of work, interactions with other workers, uses of technologies, and taken-for-granted aspects of work.

During the ride-along observations, I informally interviewed paramedics based on what I had observed. These interviews/conversations were held during paramedics' "downtime," when they were between calls or were finishing up a call after the patient was transferred to the hospital. The duration and timing of these interview/conversations were determined by the rhythms of the paramedics' work; when a call came in, the interview was abandoned until another quiet moment on that shift or during a subsequent shift. I conducted 115 interviews in total with paramedics, with an average length of 18 minutes (range: 2.25–81 minutes).

The interviews were aimed at two analytical goals: 1) Understanding the work processes of paramedics, and 2) Eliciting talk from paramedics about how their work connects or hooks up with institutional relations that structure their work and make their work processes visible. I would typically ask paramedics to explain to me what they did, why they did it, and how they knew what to do. I would also ask many clarification questions. For example, if I noticed that paramedics said something in relation to the Dispatch Centre or Emergency Department or did something with a medical or knowledge technology that was new to me or that I did not understand, I would ask them to explain it to me. Many of my questions to paramedics were oriented towards understanding how what they did was written up in the electronic patient care record and other technologies, and how their work interfaced with other institutional sites.

As observations and interviews unfolded, I began to ask paramedics about some of their "tricks of the trade," a question that was geared towards understanding "how and what they learned [and did] outside formal processes" (Smith, 2005, p. 139). In order to better understand the tensions paramedics face on the front lines of emergency health services, I asked participants to talk about or to indicate "the times you are frustrated" (Rankin, personal communication). Because I wanted to have a well-rounded understanding of paramedics' work, and the context in which their work occurs, I also listened for and asked questions about what was working well for paramedics. My goal in observing and interviewing paramedics was to gain a better understanding of what they do and the organizational site in which that work took place.

While I began in the everyday work of paramedics, I did not stop there; institutional ethnographers typically seek to move beyond description of local events to explicate how what people do is shaped by institutional relations of coordination and control. Therefore, this research also explores how the work of paramedics connects to and is organized by other individuals *off the streets* in EMS. To do so, I investigated the work of other key players in EMS, including emergency department physicians and nurses, EMS supervisors and administrators, and other individuals integral to the function of the emergency medical system, such as call-takers and dispatchers. In addition to interviewing these individuals, I observed the work of Dispatch Centre workers and the work of an acting paramedic supervisor.

Interviews during this phase of the research were semi-structured and organized around a small set of topics generated from my observations of paramedics' work. The focus of these interviews was to gain a better understanding of the way EMS is organized and monitored. When talking to these participants, I asked questions about how their work connected to the work of paramedics on the street and how this connection was made. Because IE views texts and different technologies as *active* in people's everyday lives and central to how lives are governed (Campbell & Gregor, 2002, p. 22), I also asked questions about the different texts and text-based technologies they used, what type of information was collected (what information was counted), how this information was used and made visible and to whom, and how this information impacted their work. Furthermore, I spoke with these individuals about any tension that arose in their work and how this tension was connected with the work of others. Through these questions, this phase explored how health and government administrative organizations enter into and mediate paramedics' work processes (Rankin & Campbell, 2006).

In total, I conducted 36 interviews in this phase, half of which occurred in the Dispatch Centre. The interviews lasted, on average, 53 minutes. Dispatch Centre personnel whom I interviewed included call-takers, dispatchers, managers of call-takers and dispatchers, and managers of the Dispatch Centre. For the other 18 interviews, I interviewed two managers of paramedics (one was an acting manager) and their manager, two medical directors (emergency room physicians), two individuals responsible for performance management and improvement, two teaching and learning specialists and their manager, an individual who worked closely with the electronic patient care record, an individual who worked closely with the Regional Emergency Patient Access and Coordination system, two triage nurses, and three people who worked in EMS simulation (one of whom was interviewed twice).

Overview of Book – Summary of Chapters

Part 1 of the book consists of four chapters that provide a complex, extended ethnographic examination into the everyday work of paramedics. Similar to Diamond (1992), I draw from a compilation of observations and interviews with paramedics during my ride-alongs and weave them together to tell a story that provides readers with an understanding of what paramedics do – a central theme throughout this book. Each of these chapters is constructed around an ethnographic description of one shift. I use Jake, Julie, Hanna, and Dan (pseudonyms) as the primary characters throughout these chapters. While the content that is used throughout these chapters is directly based on calls that I observed and interviews with paramedics, the accounts I provide are not attributed to any one paramedic or observation because I draw on the entirety of my data (all of the observations and interviews I conducted) to construct each composite shift. The accounts given and the characters described should therefore be viewed as composite.

The use of composite characters and ethnographic descriptions protected the anonymity of participants by making it difficult for people to identify those who participated in this study from the observations I describe and the words of participants I use. Furthermore, these composite accounts and characters allowed me to draw on a diversity of interviews and observations and to represent complex stories about work processes that show "what I learned" (Campbell & Gregor, 2002, p. 93) as aligned with the analytical goal of this research – to draw attention to some of the complexities of what paramedics do, and how what they do is socially organized, counted, and made institutionally visible. The compilations also draw attention to what counts for paramedics; as will be discussed later, often what counts for paramedics is contrary to what counts institutionally.

In chapter 2, I introduce readers to Jake and Julie, both of whom are Emergency Medical Technicians-Paramedics (EMT-Ps), and their practicum student named April. I use this chapter to set the scene, so to speak, by introducing readers to the paramedic station, the ambulance unit, and some of the medical tools and technologies paramedics use. After setting the scene, I take readers on a call, where we see Jake and Julie in action. In chapter 3, I introduce readers to another crew, Hanna and Dan, both of whom are EMT-Ps. I take readers on a heart-wrenching "hospital relief" call where Hanna and Dan come into contact with an aboriginal patient who is "parked" in the hallway of the hospital waiting for a bed to become available. In chapter 4, I take readers on another shift with Jake and Julie. This chapter builds on the previous chapters by drawing attention to additional complexities of paramedics' work. I conclude part 1 with chapter 5, where I provide an epilogue about my observations and analyses discussed in chapters 2–4.

In part 2 of this book, I provide an in-depth look into sites of coordination and governance central to contemporary emergency medical services. In these chapters, I bring to the fore institutional technologies that are central to how the work of paramedics is structured and made institutionally visible and which play a key role in health care reform practices. In chapter 6, I focus on the work of people in the Dispatch Centre – call-takers, dispatchers, and their managers – and ethnographically explore how the work of these individuals connects to the front-line work of paramedics and the institutional processes central to this interface. I also focus on different institutional technologies central to this work setting. In chapter 7, I explore additional technologies in EMS, such as the medical protocols and electronic patient care record, that are geared towards targeting and taming clinical practices and producing knowledge of paramedics' work practices. These technologies intersect with the technologies discussed in chapter 6 and play an integral role in quality improvement and quality assurance projects that are increasingly targeting front-line EMS work.

I conclude this book with chapter 8, where I provide an in-depth discussion that critically examines the work of pre-hospital health care professionals in the age of technological governance. I revisit the hidden dangers that were described in the ethnographic chapters and discuss the need to address governance practices organized by discourses of neoliberalism, accountability, and efficiency. It is in this light that I extend the findings of this book and discuss its broader implications. I also discuss how this book and, more generally, this type of research offer empirical evidence that "talks back" to conventional health services research and the type of knowledge used to reform health care systems and front-line work.

PART ONE

Chapter Two

Setting the Scene

The Station

Today I am riding with Jake and Julie, both of whom are EMT-Ps with about 10 years and five years of experience as paramedics respectively. It is 6:00 in the morning, 30 minutes before the official start of the shift. Paramedics at this station, and this is a common practice with the other crews I observed, arrive for their shifts half an hour early in order to allow the crew they are replacing to leave on time, just in case a call comes in during the last 30 minutes of their shift. It is a small station with a garage that can fit two ambulances. I enter through a side door, which leads into a short hallway that opens up into a television room with an armchair and two three-person couches. The kitchen, located next to the TV room, has a refrigerator, sink, stove and oven, cupboards, and a table that sits six people. Also in the station are two bathrooms and two bedrooms. Each bedroom has two twin-size cots with a divider between them. Throughout my ride-alongs, I learned that paramedics do not usually have time to use the bedrooms and frequently get interrupted when using the kitchen.

This is a stand-alone station, which means the paramedics do not share it with fire department personnel, as is the case with some other stations in the city. In Calgary, there are different "platoons" that rotate in the hall to provide 24-hours-a-day, seven-days-a-week coverage at each station. For the most part, paramedics in Calgary work consecutive two-day shifts and two-night shifts that are 12 hours long each, followed by four days off. In addition, some stations have more than two crews who can have overlapping shifts, which have been introduced during peak times to alleviate system "pressures."

As I enter the building, I say hello to Julie, who is reclining in the armchair, polishing her boots. She says in a calm and reassuring voice, "It's going to be a good day today. Someone's going to die." She explains to me that whenever she polishes her boots, someone dies. I think to myself, why would she be polishing her boots then? Perhaps she wanted me to see a "good" call. Soon after I arrive, Jake enters the station, his big personality already blaring. I say hi to Jake and he says something along the lines of "not you again." I laugh, and he satirically looks at me with a stone-cold face. Both paramedics are in attire that would be typical of all of my ride-alongs: dark blue pants, heavy jackets with "EMS" logos stitched on their shirts, leather boots, and thick black belts. A few minutes after Jake arrives, a young-looking woman arrives. As she enters the building, Jake jokingly says, "You're late, Stu."

"Stu" is the name given to April because she is Jake and Julie's student, who, as part of her EMT training, is riding with them for a few weeks. This part of April's training is considered her practicum and occurs near the end of EMT and EMT-P training programs. The goal of a practicum is for students to apply knowledge learned in school to a real-life work environment, and to learn from more experienced paramedics, known as preceptors. According to Julie, this teaching work is done for "free" by both preceptors and students. Julie explains her teaching work as follows:

> We're teaching them the basics; the things that we're not thinking of anymore. Assessments, patient contact, differential diagnosis ... It's harder to teach because I forget that you have to learn patient assessment and that you have to learn the basic things.

Jake explains it a bit differently: he does not teach students "what to think" per se but "how to think. To think through and solve this problem ... I don't care what you learned in school. How are you going to rationalize it in a high-stress situation? How are you going to sit [act and react] through the call?"

Four of my other ride-alongs also had students. Two of these crews had the students leading some calls in their entirety, or parts of a call. In both scenarios, the preceptors closely supervised the students by staying close to them and listening carefully while they were attending to a patient. The other two crews had the students primarily observing the work of the paramedics. The latter scenario was the case for my observations with Jake, Julie, and April.

I found these ride-alongs with students particularly interesting because the paramedics would often coach and explain to the student what they were looking for in terms of how the student should interact with and treat the patient. Sometimes the preceptors would ask their students to answer medically and institutionally relevant questions in a quizzing fashion. This teaching work inevitably exemplified some of the thinking behind paramedics' work processes. The students I observed also carried with them a booklet where they practised doing patient care reports (PCRs) based on the calls they led or observed. April explained to me that Jake and Julie would review the reports with her and tell her the things she needed to work on. She also explained that as her practicum progresses, the skills that she is expected to demonstrate, as made visible in the report, will change based on certain competencies. At the end of the practicum, the reports will be evaluated by her preceptor – "I have to reference which PCRs that I achieved these competencies and then I have to get them to sign off on it." The preceptor gives a final appraisal of the student's performance, with the power to pass or fail the student. This assessment carries significant weight in the training program; if the student fails her practicum, she may not pass the program. While Jake expects his students to be "dumb" when they do their practicum because they are "not going to know the job," what he looks for at the end of the practicum is whether or not a student can "stumble through a call" and "not kill" somebody; "do they meet the minimum?"[1]

Jake and Julie were the only crew to refer to their student as "Stu," though it was not the first time I heard paramedics refer to each other by nicknames, and I would not be surprised if such nicknames were used by other paramedics in reference to their students. Jake and Julie, for example, had nicknames for each other that were made up from parts of their last names. They used those nicknames in endearing ways throughout my observations of them. We might view this reference to April as "Stu" as a term of endearment that signalled that she belonged to the team or was being initiated into the EMS team. On the other hand, "Stu" is a very generic word that is void of any individual signifiers and might be considered objectifying and homogenizing. Seen this way, the linguistic turn to refer to April as "Stu" might symbolize that April has not yet been accepted into the culture of EMS and thus must go through this rite of passage and/or initiation process in order to gain acceptance and truly become a member of the team. Lastly, naming April "Stu" can also be seen as socially organized, connected to regulations of training, evaluation, and institutional expectations of mentorship.

The Ambulance

Soon after April arrives, I follow Jake, Julie, and April out to the garage, where the ambulance, otherwise known as the "apparatus unit," "truck," or "rig," has just arrived, probably back from a call. The paramedics in the ambulance step out and briefly speak to Jake and Julie. After a few minutes of talking, one of the paramedics gives Jake a pouch that Jake attaches to his belt. I learn later that this pouch carries certain "controlled substances" that have to be "on his person" at all times because only EMT-Ps are licensed to give these drugs (e.g., morphine). After the other crew leaves, Julie goes over to a computer mounted between the driver and passenger seat, referred to by Jake and Julie as the CAD (Computer Aided Dispatch), and enters her and Jake's paramedic registration numbers. After signing in, Julie grabs a binder from the ambulance and begins to walk around the ambulance. She explains that the binder contains the "vehicle check list" document that paramedics are supposed to fill out and sign at the beginning of each shift; signing the document signifies that certain tasks have been completed at the beginning of the shift, such as checking over the ambulance and ensuring that stocks of supplies are present in it. According to Julie, this ensures that "the vehicle is ready for our, um, string of calls." She also explains that this documentary practice is "especially [important] with Alberta Health Services [AHS]. They want to hold people more accountable. With the city [prior to reform (see chapter 1)] you could actually get away with quite a bit. It's a different story here with the provincial government, 'cause if they can pass blame, they will."

As Julie slowly circles the ambulance, I notice her opening some doors (including the hood) for a quick inspection. While doing so, she mentions that this ambulance is a newer version (discussed in chapter 3), which is not as good as the "old ones." Jake, who is in the back of the ambulance with April, yells, "They were quickly rushed in." As we continue to walk around the ambulance, intermittently stopping, Julie explains to me that it is the driver's responsibility to check over the ambulance, including its mechanics, to make sure it is street safe, whereas it is the attendant (the paramedic who leads the call) who generally checks the bags and supplies in the back of the ambulance, which is what Jake is doing.

I noticed throughout my ride-alongs that the paramedic in the passenger seat is generally the attending paramedic – the one who typically leads the call and attends to the patient. The non-attending paramedic is the one who often drives and assists the attending paramedic. I observed crews change who was leading the call and who was assisting either halfway through the shift or after every 12-hour shift. Jake and Julie preferred to switch after every shift. With that said, these separate roles are often not delineated, because they can change depending on the type and complexity of the call, and depending on the designation of paramedics. For example, only EMT-Ps can attend to Advanced Life Support or ALS calls, compared to an EMT, who can only attend to Basic Life Support or BLS calls. If an attending paramedic is an EMT and the call is classified as an ALS call, the non-attending EMT-P is supposed to take over and attend to the patient.

After quickly checking off some boxes and signing the checklist, Julie returns the binder to its place and we join Jake and April in the back of the ambulance. I sit down in the airway seat, the same seat that I would sit in throughout most of my ride-alongs,[2] and note some of the "standard" features of the ambulance. The back of the ambulance has three seats: the airway seat, which is located at the head of the stretcher and can rotate to look out the front or the back of the ambulance; the bench seat, which is about a metre in length and is typically where the attendant sits while in the back with the patient; and an additional seat opposite the bench seat that could be used for various reasons, including chest compressions. The back of the ambulance also has two doors, one at the rear that can be used when a patient is being loaded headfirst into the ambulance on the stretcher, and one at the side, which will often be used if the patient can walk with little or no assistance. Perpendicular to the bench seat and located at the side entrance of the ambulance is a net that is attached to the ceiling and ground of the unit. In addition to instructing patients to use the net when they are entering the ambulance, Julie later explained that the net would also catch a paramedic if s/he were thrown around while in the back of the ambulance.

There are cupboards throughout the ambulance with different supplies. All ambulances also have a place for a set of three bags (red, blue, and black), referred to as the "Christmas tree"; paramedics bring different combinations of these bags when they leave the ambulance. Jake explains that the red or "primary" bag is used on all calls: "as far as the rules go, you're supposed to always take in the red bag with you at all times, 'cause you never know what you have." This bag includes "your diagnostic equipment," like the blood pressure cuff, glucometer, and IV supplies. Other bags include the cardiac monitor, which "goes into

2.1 The back of the ambulance

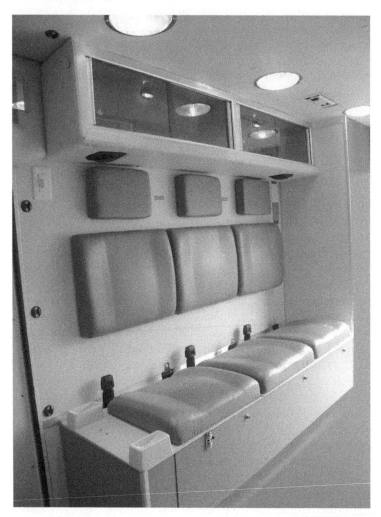

Above: the bench seat. Top, facing page: the airway seat and the net. The stretcher is typically located parallel to the bench seat on the right and is secured to the metal device located on the floor of the unit. Bottom, facing page: the third seat. In all three photos, cupboards can be seen dispersed throughout the ambulance. Images courtesy of Demers Ambulances.

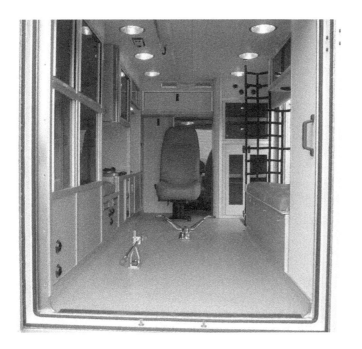

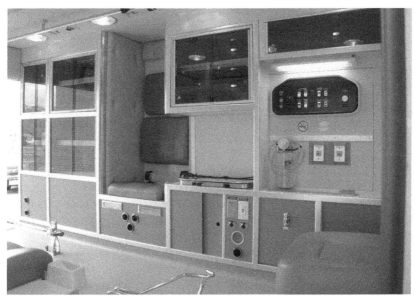

most calls too," and the airway kit, which is the third bag. Jake explains the use of the bags as follows:

> On your standard call ... I just call it one kit, two kit, or three kit call ... Let's say someone's sick, just generalized sick – it sounds like someone's been sick for a few days – I might just take the one bag with me. If it sounds like a chest pain, you bring the cardiac monitor and oxygen ... If it sounds like a possible cardiac arrest, you grab the third bag, which is the uh, airway kit.

The type of call that Jake is referring to is based primarily on the information he receives from the Dispatch Centre that appears on the CAD, which includes the "call type" and the "notes" entered by the call-taker (discussed below). While this information is important, Jake explained that he "decipher[s]" between this information provided by Dispatch and the actual settings of his work – "truthfully too, if you're going up the uh, if you're going up the high-rise apartment, a lot of time you'll throw more stuff on [the stretcher] than usual because you'll have to hike down."

Sitting in the ambulance, I watch Jake open cupboards, shuffle through the supplies, and move stuff around, intermittently pulling trays and supplies out, often putting them back immediately, though occasionally he places some of the supplies in a trash bag. He also places what I would later find out were "barf bags" in between the two pads that make up the backrest of the airway seat for quick access. While doing this, he explains to April how this preparation work at the beginning of a shift is central to how he makes the ambulance – his "office" – his own. Jake then looks at me and describes this part of his preparation work as "titrating" the ambulance "based on how we practise our medicine." Julie adds that some paramedics like to have enough stock on an ambulance to "do calls [for], you know, an entire week without ... stocking up." Julie, on the other hand, "hate[s] clutter and I find it often gets in the way and it makes it more difficult to keep a truck orderly." As she says this, Julie begins to "pull" some of the "clutter" left by the previous crew – "we have five bags of saline in here. That's ridiculous. We don't need that many." Julie, while looking at me and intermittently turning away to look at April, goes on to explain that titrating the ambulance depends on the day of the week; they "overstock" on supplies depending on the type of calls they expect to have on the day of the week and the time of year. On Friday and Saturday nights, for example, "we're going to need our cannulas[3] there.

That will be a big thing. Why? Drunks, accidents, all that type of stuff."
Julie goes on:

> When weekends come, you know, you're gonna get ready for traumas
> and stuff like that. You know, fights, so you've got to make sure all your
> dressings, you got enough of that kicking around. Saline so you can wash
> people's eyes out 'cause somebody will get pepper sprayed.

As Julie explains this to April and me, I notice Jake placing what
looks like a boom-box device that says "Lifepak" on it near the end of
the bench seat, opposite a mount that I later find out is meant to hold
this medical device in place. After moving the Lifepak, Jake turns to me
and tells me that this is "one of the most important things on the rig."
He explains to me that the Lifepak is a multi-purpose medical device
that can measure a patient's blood pressure and oxygen levels and con-
duct ECGs, and can be used as a defibrillator when necessary. To finish
their preparations, Jake places a makeshift trashcan made from a plastic
container in between the net and the bench seat.

The Tones

No longer than 15 minutes after preparing the ambulance, I hear
what the paramedics refer to as the tones, a loud, piercing alarm that,
throughout over 200 hours of observations with paramedics, always
jolted me from whatever I was doing. This tone, sent to our station
by the Dispatch Centre, indicates that we have a call. Jake and Julie
quickly stop what they are doing and put the supplies away. Jake hops
into the front passenger seat of the ambulance while Julie hops into the
driver's seat. April secures herself in the bench seat. Facing forward
in the airway seat, I see Julie press a button on the dashboard and
glance at the CAD. I notice that Jake and Julie seem upset. According
to the CAD, the call for the paramedics is to attend to an individual
experiencing problems with his catheter. Is this a "bad call," I think to
myself? No longer than two minutes after being toned, we leave the
station. While we are slowly driving out of the garage, Jake picks up
his radio attached to the CAD, presses a button, and acknowledges to
Dispatch that they are in the ambulance and responding to the call:
"Dispatch, 210 responding to an Alpha 26." 210 refers to the unit's
number and Alpha is the call type. Alpha is the least severe call type,
a non-emergency or "cold" response without lights and sirens. 26 is

known as the "card type" of the call as determined by the Dispatch Centre. This determination is facilitated by an internationally used standardized rolodex system that categorizes information between the call-taker at the Dispatch Centre and the individual who phoned 911 (discussed in chapter 6). A card 26 refers to a "sick person." This is a very broad and general classification that one paramedic described as "the catch all" card that many of the calls I observed were categorized as. While on the way to the scene, I notice sounds coming from the CAD; after every sound, Jake immediately looks at the CAD, presses a button, and reads what appears to be an update from the Dispatch Centre about the call.

While Julie is driving, Jake explains to April and me in a loud voice how he garners and filters through the information from the CAD and how this information organizes his work. He explains how the call type will often determine whether they drive lights and sirens (hot) or not (all call types except for Alpha are hot responses). Jake goes on to explain how the call type might impact his initial reaction to the call; if the call was an Echo, he might "get excited"; however, if it is an Alpha call, and, as in this example, a card 26, he thinks to himself, "this [call] might suck." He explains that he takes all of the information from the Dispatch Centre "with a grain of salt" because "most people have no idea what an actual emergency is. So even when it sounds really bad, it's generally not." He qualifies this statement by stressing that there are "plenty of times that you'll show up and the problem has absolutely nothing to do with what actually came up [on the CAD]." What is important, according to Jake, are the "notes" that the people in the Dispatch Centre add to the call that appears on the CAD while en route. He explains that "good" dispatchers will use their experience to pass on relevant information to paramedics, like "something's weird in the background … It sounds like there's some chaos in the background." After Jake explains this to April and me, April turns to me and in a quiet voice whispers, "You learn not to trust Dispatch."

About 10 minutes after being dispatched, we arrive at the address provided by the CAD and quickly get out of the unit. Jake grabs the red bag and throws it over his shoulder while Julie grabs the Lifepak and what looks like a laptop computer, known as the electronic Patient Care Record (ePCR). Julie, April, and I follow behind Jake, who walks up a set of steps to the front door of a single-story house, maybe built in the 1960s or 1970s. He knocks on the door, which is slightly ajar, and announces in a loud voice that EMS is here. We walk right into the house and are directed by someone who I assume is the landlady to a room. I assume this because she is of a different ethnicity from the patient, as I would later find out, and she does not express concern about the patient in the way I would expect from a family member. Jake knocks on the door to the room and slowly opens it. As he enters the room, he introduces himself as a paramedic to the individual resting on a mattress on the floor. Julie follows Jake into the room, and April and I follow closely behind.

Positioned near the door, I notice immediately the smell and lay-out of the room. It smells like stale air with dirt and mould or mildew mixed in. The room is about 8 by 10 feet in size and has a twin mattress placed on the floor, a stained dark green carpet, a TV placed on the floor in the corner of the room, a closet with one change of clothes hanging from the hanger, and a small – about three by one foot in length – table located next to the bed with an open can of what seems like a tomato-based food of some type. The patient is an adult male who looks much older than the 55 years of age that he tells Jake he is. He is very skinny, to the point where I write in my fieldnotes "malnourished"; he does not have any fat on his body, and his facial bones are clearly protruding from his face.

Assessment Work – "We're Trying to Play a Chess Match, Three, Five Moves Ahead"

Jake approaches the patient and asks him for his health care card. The patient shifts his body, reaches into his pocket and pulls out a thin wallet, opens it and produces a card that he hands to Jake. Jake quickly hands the card to Julie, who then opens the ePCR, which is like a small laptop computer, and begins to enter information into the tablet while Jake, in a calm and relaxed voice, starts to ask the patient some questions. "My friend, what is the problem?" The patient places his hand gently on his stomach and says in a soft and mumbling voice that he is having pain. Jake asks the patient to lift up his shirt and gently places his hand on the patient's stomach and applies pressure. As Jake presses, the patient lets out a painful moan. Jake quickly removes his hand and asks, "You taking any medications? Do you smoke?"[4]

While Jake is talking to the patient, Julie unzips a pouch attached to the Lifepak and takes out a set of wires. At the end of the wires are electrodes that can be attached to the patient's body. Julie assists Jake in placing these around the patient's pectoral muscles, the sides of the chest, and the lower part of each leg. Once the electrodes are attached, Jake presses a button on the Lifepak, and after about one minute, a long strip of paper emerges from the machine. Jake and Julie later explain to me that this technology can be used to "take a picture of the heart," known as an electrocardiogram (ECG), and provide a printout of this picture. To my untrained eye, the picture looks like a bunch of squiggly lines.

In between placing the electrodes on the patient's body and reading the printout from the Lifepak, Jake places a blood pressure cuff, which is also connected to the Lifepak, around the patient's arm. With the press of a button on the front of the Lifepak, the cuff inflates and produces some numbers that are displayed on the front of the Lifepak. Julie also connects a little attachment from the Lifepak to the patient's index finger to measure what I would later find out were his oxygen levels. While Jake is speaking to the patient, I notice that he glances at the number on the Lifepak out of the corner of his eye. Next, I notice Julie taking out a thermometer from the red bag and swiping it across and down the side of the patient's forehead and briefly showing the number to Jake.

After Jake has assessed the patient for about 10 minutes, Julie leaves the room and heads outside to the ambulance while Jake stays with the patient. April and I follow Julie. No more than a 10-metre walk from the house, we arrive at the ambulance, and Julie unbuckles the seatbelts from the stretcher, adjusts the sheets and pillow, and takes out an IV bag full of fluids from one of the cupboards in the unit and places it next to her on the bench seat. She also takes out a roll of tape, tears off a few pieces, and places them on the backrest of the bench seat. While doing this preparation work, Julie takes out an orange book located in her vest pocket and quickly opens it, flips to her desired page, and looks at the page for about 30 seconds.

While she is prepping the ambulance, I ask Julie to explain what happened in the house. She explains that Jake did a medical assessment of the patient. She goes on to explain that the assessments paramedics do are based primarily on the biomedical training that they receive in school. She explains this by discussing a call that she attended the day before, when a patient was experiencing chest pain:

> In medicine you do what's a primary survey and then you do a secondary survey or a focused survey. So a primary survey is when I look at you, sick or not sick. Are you pink? Are you working hard to breathe? The very, very basic picture of our patient ... And then after that you either go to

a focused exam, in this case I did a focused exam trying to figure out if this is cardiac or not. So I'm asking her a lot of questions about her chest discomfort and where it's moving to 'cause she said it was moving up her jaw and stuff like that. Sometimes after you've done a primary, you still have no clue what's going on so instead of doing a focused exam you end up doing what's called a secondary exam and you're literally going from head to toe on a patient and you're trying to find stuff. Sometimes you won't find stuff.

She goes on to talk about how assessments vary depending on the nature of the call; some calls are more traumatic in nature, therefore you "treat what you see," whereas other calls, like this one, are more "medical in nature," which often requires more investigation (see Nurok & Henckes, 2009). Based on all of the information garnered through the initial assessment, including the information produced through medical devices, which she explains can be used to "trend" the patient, paramedics can arrive at a chief complaint and a "working diagnosis." I ask Julie if this connects in some way to the orange book she briefly took out and looked at, and she replies that it does because the chief complaint can determine what protocols and treatments are followed and applied to the patient. Such protocols, she goes on, are located in the orange book.[5]

Julie is quick to point out that assessment work is not as straightforward as she just described it; while initial information is "acted upon," assessment work is continuous and is based on the unfolding of "remarkable" information (Corman, 2016). Julie provides the metaphor of driving down a road to exemplify this work process. While she may begin by "going west" on a road, depending on new and emerging information – "and you're constantly, literally navigating through and reacting to the environment and the situation as it is" – her direction might change and she might "merge" or "branch off" and go "another way." Referring back to "trending" the patient, she speaks about the constant need to assess the patient "to show that they're always on this level and they're not getting any better and they're not getting worse." She exemplifies how this mental work orients and reorients to a continuous flow of information based on answers from questions asked, observations made, and information garnered from the medical devices.

Julie gives an example of continuous assessment work by referring back to a previous call I had observed her and Jake on when they attended to a pedestrian who was hit by a car. While Jake approached the driver, I followed Julie as she approached the patient, who was lying face down in the street. Julie kneeled down and began asking the patient questions. I heard the patient say, "I feel shaky." After about five minutes of speaking with the patient, Julie helped her stand up and assisted her to the ambulance. In the ambulance, Julie asked the patient, "What hurts the most now?" and she responded, "My wrist." While Julie told the patient that she might have a "fractured" wrist, Julie continued to assess the patient by placing her hands on different parts of her back and neck and asking about levels of pain as she pressed against the patient's body. As Jake began to splint the patient's arm, Julie told the patient in a stern voice, "If anything changes, you need to let me know."

After the patient was transferred to the hospital, Julie explains to me that she was initially ready to board the patient (put the patient on a hard board and secure her head, referred to as C-Spine), but then she received some additional information from Jake; "She said this and he got some information that I didn't get, then we combine information and based on that you know I can go, 'Yah we don't need to board her.'" Julie also mentions how she did a physical exam of the patient where she sat her up and checked her spine, and "clear[ed]" C-Spine. Julie goes on to explain how her decision not to "board" the patient was based on this continuous assessment work:

So I mean it's constantly flowing, and things change and things progress ... Once again, new information flowing in here, well I had to react on that first bit of information or else we'd still be on scene ... You make your decision, things change, you adapt ... I've had to board people halfway to the hospital ...

After Julie has prepped the ambulance for about five minutes, Jake arrives with the patient and assists him in through the side door. As the patient gets into the ambulance, I notice that he is breathing heavily and seems to be struggling to catch his breath. Jake tells him to lie on the stretcher whatever way is most comfortable. Suddenly, Jake and Julie's demeanour changes; the atmosphere in the unit becomes more intense and the work of the paramedics seems to speed up while silence briefly overtakes the unit. Jake quickly takes his stethoscope out of in his front vest pocket, places the ends into his ears and the flat metal piece onto the patient's chest. With his head slightly tilted, he listens while Julie presses a button on the Lifepak and takes another reading of the patient's heart activity. While Jake is still listening, Julie tears the printout away from the machine and reads it for about 20 seconds. She writes something down on the palm of one of her hands and shows it to Jake. She then shows it to me. It reads, "JVD," which stands for jugular venous distension and is associated with congestive heart failure. Julie then passes the printout to Jake, who takes a quick look and reattaches the device onto the index finger of the patient. The environment now seems more calm and relaxed. Jake takes out a small device and pricks the patient's other index finger, absorbs some of the blood with a white strip, and inserts the strip into the device to check what I later learn are the patient's blood sugar levels. Soon after, Jake suggests to the patient that he receive some oxygen to help him catch his breath and places the oxygen tubes gently over the patient's face and around his ears to secure the tubes.

"REPAC Please"

Next, Julie presses a button on the dispatch radio clipped on her shoulder and says, "8 code 15. REPAC please." Dispatch quickly responds, though I cannot discern what they say. Julie then exits from the back of the ambulance and goes to the driver's seat while Jake sits on the bench seat and opens the ePCR. April and I secure ourselves in our seats and we leave for the hospital. REPAC, I would later discover, is a relatively new technology geared towards improving the "flow" of the EMS and emergency departments in Calgary. To do so, REPAC categorizes each hospital into a green (not so busy), yellow (getting busy), or red (busy) status based on a multiplicity of data, as will be discussed in chapter 6. The technology "recommends" to the crew, via the dispatcher, the most "appropriate" hospital to transport the patient to, based on its colour-coded status. Typically, the green status is recommended. I asked Jake and Julie if REPAC works well, and Julie replied, "works on paper, not always in real life" (further discussed in later chapters).

On the way to the hospital, I notice that Jake positions his body while sitting on the bench seat towards the patient and continues talking to him. While chatting with the patient, Jake also intermittently taps on the ePCR, which is open in front of him and resting on his lap. I notice him asking the patient additional questions that seem to be related to demographic information and past medical history. Jake later explained that the questions he was asking were primarily geared towards filling out sections of the ePCR, as he put it, "for their care." While asking these questions he also begins to, what I began to think of as, "shoot the shit" with the patient by telling self-deprecating but jovial jokes. For Jake, much of this "shooting the shit" work is to let his patients know that "we haven't forgotten about them [and] to ease them and possibly distract them." Jake went on to explain:

> It's to keep their mind off of the issue and you can see, they're starting to smile, their heart rate is going down, their blood pressures come down. I'm having an effect here. I'm having a physiological effect on this patient here. I'm able to calm him down and that's, that's kind of a big thing we do in our job, we usually get to the chaotic scene [and] you have to bring back calmness and order there and get everybody back to normal if you can. Calming them is part of your reassessment.

In addition to shooting the shit with this patient, Jake does some teaching work on the way to the hospital by trying to inform the patient of the services that are available in Calgary. The patient, for example, tells Jake that he cannot afford his medications. Jake explains that there are some services available to assist him in paying for them.

The Hospital

We arrive at the hospital about 25 minutes after leaving the scene. According to Dispatch, the hospital we were REPACed to was the least busy hospital in Calgary. As we enter the ambulance garage bay, I notice there are two ambulances already parked in the garage. After the ambulance stops, Julie exits from her seat in the front, walks around to the back, opens the door, and with her left hand pushes a lever, which detaches the stretcher from its locked position. Jake jumps down through the rear of the ambulance and assists Julie in unloading the stretcher. As the patient is being unloaded from the unit, an additional ambulance rolls into the garage. Julie pushes the stretcher and follows Jake, who is a few feet ahead of her with the ePCR in hand. April and I follow. We walk through a long hallway and two minutes later arrive at the triage desk.

Triage is an area in the hospital that is responsible for assessing the acuity of patients, whether they walk into the emergency department (ED) or are brought in by EMS. Pam, a triage nurse whom I interviewed, describes her work as follows:

So being a triage nurse your job is to, you know, do a quick assessment of the patient that's come up to the window, find out what they're there for, and determine … how sick they are. So, we do a set of vital signs, we do a quick … assessment like airway, breathing, [and] circulation … If it's a chest pain or shortness of breath we'll listen to their chest, we'll listen to their heart sounds, we'll do a quick set of vitals and determine, you know, OK is this patient in cardiac, is this patient having breathing problems, you know, if not, then they can go to a non-monitored area, and if we're concerned about them then we have the CTAS [Canadian Triage and Acuity Scale] system to … categorize our patients … [and] figure out the priority.

One of the primary roles of a triage nurse is to allocate resources in the ED by determining who needs to be seen by a physician the soonest. The allocation of ED space follows accordingly.

Once we arrive at triage, Jake places the stretcher holding the patient against the wall and approaches the triage nurse, who is sitting behind a counter with three computers in front of her. I would later learn that two of the computers are dedicated to triaging patients; one is for walk-in patients and one is for patients brought in by EMS.[6] The third computer is "our REDIS [Regional Emergency Department Information Systems] computer system,"[7] which, according to the triage nurse, is "a computer system, so it tracks the patients in the department" and acts as a map of the resources available, like which beds are being cleaned, occupied by patients, and available for new patients. I notice on the REDIS computer that there is a bright green bar on the screen, which I later learn means that the hospital is not in any alert and that space should theoretically be available.

Information about the patient (e.g., Who is he? What brought him to the emergency department? What treatments were given? What is his blood pressure reading?) is passed along in what seems like a brief encounter between Jake and the triage nurse. Next, Jake takes a few steps back and stands behind the stretcher. Another individual, who I would later learn is the admitting clerk, approaches Jake. Jake opens the ePCR, and the person takes a quick look at the device and then walks away. Soon after, the triage nurse prints off a piece of paper entitled the "Emergency Assessment and Treatment Record" and hands it to Jake. The patient is quickly placed into a room near the triage station where Julie assists him in taking off his clothes and putting on a gown. While Julie is assisting the patient, Jake walks over to someone, who I would later learn is the unit nurse assigned to our patient, gives her the piece of paper that was handed to him by the triage nurse, and begins to speak to the nurse quietly.

I later asked Jake what he said to the triage and unit nurses. What follows, and this resonates with most if not all of the paramedics I spoke with, is how he described his thinking behind what he and other paramedics referred to as "giving report." He characterized the information he gave the triage nurse as the "Cole's Notes" or abbreviated version of the call; "what we've found – all the major stuff that's going to affect the decision as to where they're [the triage nurse] going to put them [the patient] … I'm going to tell you exactly what you need to know so that you can make a quick decision as to where you want to put the patient or if you want us to hold on to the patient and wait in the hallway … Um, that's kind of the trust … because they're basing their decision on what we're, on our assessment …" Jake compared the Cole's Notes version of events to what he tells the unit nurse once the patient is transferred to a unit in the hospital, which is more "detailed"; he "tell[s] them everything that you know that is pertinent. If it's not pertinent then you don't tell them." In other words, the triage nurse generally gets "one little blip" about the chief complaint and the relevant patient symptoms, and the unit nurse gets a "wider" story. With that said, I noticed during one ride-along that Julie stayed at the triage desk for a longer time than I had been accustomed to. I asked her to talk about this and she explained that some triage nurses "like the bigger stories but some of them just don't really care … So you kind of get to know your audience."

I am amazed by how fast this transfer happened, considering past media accounts and general discourse I had been accustomed to hearing and reading of paramedics being "parked" with their patients in the hospital (usually in a hallway designated for EMS crews and their patients) waiting for a bed to become available. When paramedics bring a patient to the hospital, it is only when the patient is officially "transferred" to the hospital that the patient becomes the legal responsibility of the hospital. In other words, if a bed is not available when the paramedic arrives and/or there are more acute "walk in" patients in the waiting room, the triage nurse can "park" the patient with the paramedic in the hallway until space in the ED becomes available. I mention my surprise at seeing this fast transfer to Jake and he tells me that he and Julie have good rapport with the triage nurses at this hospital. This statement seems consistent with his ability to make many of the nurses he comes into contact with in this ED laugh, despite what appears to be a rather tense, serious, and fast-paced environment. In fact, the REPAC system, which is connected to REDIS, seems to be eroding or displacing some of this work; in the process of "better" using hospital and EMS resources, and hence achieving the goal of better "flow," crews are sometimes diverted away from the closest hospital to the more "appropriate" one, sometimes across town. In doing so, paramedics may be directed to hospitals where they are not used to attending and have yet to develop or utilize this rapport that Jake so aptly demonstrates. Furthermore, patients may be brought to hospitals away from their local settings and social support, despite sometimes requesting a hospital they prefer.

After the patient is transferred, we all walk back through the long hallway, and Julie and April hop into the back of the ambulance and begin cleaning it while Jake sits in the front seat with the ePCR open on his lap and begins to do his "paper work." I watch as Julie and April thoroughly wipe down all of the equipment that was used on the call and dispose of any trash. As they are wiping down the ambulance, I think about how this transfer process points to a multiplicity of relations, some of which connect to the allocation of hospital resources, that organize and coordinate not only the work of paramedics but also the work of patients; rather than paramedics simply dropping off their patients at the hospital, once paramedics enter the hospital site, there are overlapping legal, medical, and other regulatory relations organizing the transfer of patients into the hospital. Once everything is disinfected in the unit, Julie walks to a set of large cupboards located against one of the walls in the garage, grabs some supplies, and brings them back to the ambulance.

While cleaning, Julie intermittently speaks with other paramedics in the garage. I hear her mention "new protocols," followed by "Don't get caught." I later learned that she was chatting with another paramedic about the new protocols that had been introduced two weeks prior to the beginning of my research. Julie and this paramedic speak for a few minutes. While I cannot hear what they are discussing, when Julie returns to the ambulance, she says to me, "We have questions every day about protocols ... they can be interpreted in different ways." It was in the context of this observation that I recalled an earlier conversation with Jake when he explained the teaching work paramedics do among themselves – "What did you guys do 'cause I was faced with a similar situation?" – where they talk to each other about their work because, as Jake explained, "We're at best teaching ourselves."

The ePCR

While Jake is sitting in the front passenger seat of the ambulance working on the ePCR, I walk over to him and look over his shoulder. I ask him to talk to me about what he is doing and he explains in depth how he enters information about the call into the ePCR. He begins by explaining that the ePCR is a newly introduced technology (around 2008) that replaced the previous paper-based version. It is used to record specific information about the call. Once the information is collected, it gets printed off and handed to the unit nurse that the patient was transferred to and put into the patient's chart. Jake also mentions that the ePCR gets uploaded onto a server and goes to EMS headquarters. In addition to collecting patient information, Jake says the ePCR is used for "auditing" purposes, which happens "periodically just to see if we're doing the right treatments on scene."

I notice that on the ePCR screen, there are different tabs available for entering information. The top horizontal row of the computer screen has the following dropdown menus: File, Window, Help, Comments, and Filters. There is also a vertical row with different tabs. When the tabs are touched, the screen goes to those tabs and all of the relevant boxes in the tabs become visible. Furthermore, with each vertical tab, there are corresponding horizontal tabs that appear once the vertical tab is pressed. Vertical tabs include ID (the patient's ID), Hx (patient history), PS (Primary Survey), V/S (Vitals), Tx (Treatment), T (Transport), R (Review). It looks something like what appears in figure 2.2.

As he clicks through the ePCR, Jake explains that it consists of many tabs and many fields within each tab. "There's certain things that need to be filled in, like for billing and that. Required fields ... For us the least important is [*laugh*] billing information." Some of the information, like the billing information, is often collected by the non-attending paramedic. Jake explains that when he gave Julie the patient's health care card, it was because the ePCR requires this information. If certain required fields are not filled in, an "override" notice will appear before you can submit the ePCR and require you to fill it in or provide an explanation as to why you did not fill it in.

The first section I see Jake filling in is under the ID tab, where he records the patient's chief complaint, which is the "main reason why

2.2 ePCR tablet (top) and screenshot (bottom)

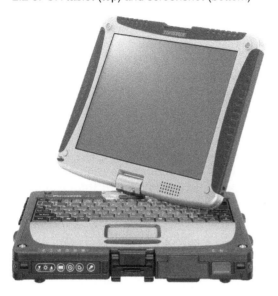

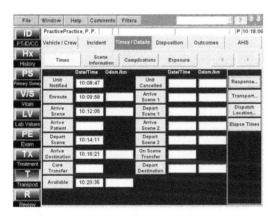

Source: ePCR Training Manual, © 2014 Alberta Health Services. See Acknowledgments for further attribution and disclaimer. An older version of Siren ePCR (v3) was in use circa September 2011. The image is used with the permission of Medusa Medical Technologies Inc. To see the most current version of the Siren ePCR suite of solutions, visit www.medusamedical.com. The image is used by kind permission of Medusa Medical Technologies Inc. Photograph of the Toughbook 19 from http://business.panasonic.com/

[the patient] called today." The chief complaint, he explains, connects to many of the other sections and categories of the ePCR. After filling out the chief complaint, he begins filling out the "history" tab. In this tab, he records information that is relevant to the chief complaint, including the "symptoms [the patient] has right now." He talks about different boxes he could select as symptoms by either tapping on them from the list provided, and "it goes yellow, that's a symptom," or tapping on the symptom twice, and a line will go through the symptom, which means the symptom is recorded as a "pertinent negative – we would expect to see that [as related to the chief complaint] but we don't." He explains that pertinent negatives and pertinent positives connect to whether the information they garner throughout the call is "remarkable" or "unremarkable," language I heard Julie use time and time again. Jake explains that recording pertinent positives and pertinent negatives is important for accountability purposes; recording them recognizes, "Yeah, I looked there but I didn't see anything. So if I didn't check anything off, it's like I didn't look at it. Right, so I want to make sure, if we went to court and they say, 'How did you not see the massive whatever on his chest?' … It's pretty much unremarkable."

On the "past medical history" tab, Jake records "any medication" the patient is on (sometimes this information is also filled in by the non-attending paramedic), and "social family history," which is a category "that we don't always fill out 'cause a lot of the time there's not a real need for it." Using the patient we just transported to the hospital as an example, Jake says that in the social family history category, he included the fact that he was not sure if the patient was getting the care that he needed at home.

After going through the patient's history, Jake moves on to the "assessment times." As he is tapping through this section, he explains that he sometimes has to "fudge this a little bit" because "when I got on scene, I didn't have [the ePCR] with me, my partner was using it when I first walked up to him [so] I don't have an assessment time." In talking about how he compensates for this, he discusses the surveillance of time and how it is recorded on the front line. "As soon as a call comes in," he says, "a call is generated on the call-taker's thing [referring to the call-takers' computer at the Dispatch Centre] … As soon as a call is picked up, the clock starts." For example, the "chute time" is the time it takes a crew to respond to a call once they are toned out; in order to stop the clock after the tones are activated, Julie pressed a button on the dashboard. Jake explains, "We have our 90 seconds from the time the bells go for us to be en route to the call. That is a watched time." In addition to the chute time, there are other times that get counted by the Dispatch Centre and then uploaded into the ePCR. Jake and Julie (who is still in the back of the ambulance but clearly listening in on our conversation) simultaneously list off other times that are tracked: "call taken, notified, dispatched, en route, arrived [at scene], transport [to hospital], transport arrived [at hospital], and then cleared [the hospital]." By looking at his arrival time, for example, he can "fudge" the time of his assessment of the patient – "we arrived on scene at 7:06 so it probably took us you know however many minutes it took us to get up there so, we'll say we arrived at him at seven [*pause*] nine. So 7:09 will be my assessment time, right."

As Jake explains to me the ePCR and his work of filling it out, a paramedic whom I do not know approaches us and asks, "Does this make you want to kill yourself?" Following this statement by the passing paramedic, Jake begins to talk about how the ePCR compares to the paper-based PCRs that came before it; the PCR was "basically almost a free format where um, you can convey a lot more," but the ePCR results in having to "pigeonhole" patients into the tick boxes, which is "one of the things I don't like about the ePCRs … 'cause this is more stats. These are geared towards statistics so everything is yes/no, yes/no, black/white, you know what I mean. It doesn't work as well in this field … The numbers don't always say everything … But, everybody will tell you it is what it is." From the back of the ambulance, Julie passionately elaborates:

When I pulled the blankets away the smell of rotting flesh and feces [came] up from under the door. When I opened the door there was granny who's obviously very emaciated in a room … And that stuff doesn't show up in the little tab … that's what has to go into the narrative.

To compensate for this pigeonhole effect of the ePCR, Jake adds additional information into the "narrative" or "comments" section, which to him (and most paramedics I spoke with) is the most important part of the ePCR. He uses the metaphor of "painting the picture" to describe the purpose of this section. He explains that if you just read the statistics part of the ePCR, "you would not really know what's going on. I mean you could kinda guess but you wouldn't get a good story. So that's why we write in our comments … [The narrative] is where I'm going to write a little, this is what we found. This is what [the patient] said. This is, kinda what's been going on." The goal of the comments section, he explains, is to provide "a more well-rounded story" that captures the "essence of the call." Jake gives the example of how he puts "on arrival" in the comments section of the ePCR. Whereas the ePCR has a box that captures the arrival time (when the unit arrives at the scene), Jake adds in the comments section what he sees upon arriving at the scene because "I think it paints a really good picture depending on the situation." For example, he might say, "Patient's walking towards ambulance with care worker. Gait is normal. No obvious distress or trauma." He mentions that, depending on the scenario, "you can add all that stuff to paint a much better picture of what was really going on and what possibly could have happened ... And quote unquote; when patients tell you certain things that are pertinent um, then, you can't do that anywhere else on the PCR."

As he is writing his comments, he tells me that one of the primary audiences he writes for in this section is the doctor in the ED. Using "joint pain" as the chief complaint of the patient, he gives me an example of what he would write: "Where is it? What is it? You know I'll describe it a bit more. You know it's been going on for four days. He hasn't had a fall, 'cause I know, nowhere in here [the other sections of the ePCR] does it say he's had a fall ... I'll describe when he feels the pain ... Does [the pain] go anywhere else?" He explains that the comments vary depending on the type and complexity of the call, but his goal is to "kind of tie it all together and give [the doctors] a nice picture when they read this of what's going on and what caused [the patient] to call today."

While Jake explains how the narrative section is geared towards filling in the gaps created or not captured by the categories in the ePCR for the doctors in the ED, Julie, who a few minutes prior has sat down in the driver's seat, provides another example of how she writes the narrative section of the ePCR directed to another audience. She refers back to the motor vehicle accident example where an individual was hit by a car and explains that, because she decided not to put the patient on the board (C-Spine), and in light of the triage nurse in the ED questioning her decision not to C-Spine the patient, she had to "really back up" her decision because she could get "fired" or "taken to court."

> When I write my PCR uh, especially in stuff like this – motor vehicle collisions ah, assaults, stabbings, if we go to a gunshot or something like that – this has to be completely unbiased; I don't put in my opinion whether or

not I think someone is guilty or not ... I will um, repeat what the patient saw or what witnesses saw only to um, to qualify my treatment for the patient and to paint a picture of their potential injuries ... and it discusses the mechanism of injury ... [which] is a major one[8] ... If this ever went to court and this lawyer got this PCR and read it, and it had anything partial in there that I thought, like you can't write that you thought the patient was drunk, that Mr Mike was drunk. Um, that is uh, I don't have the tools to diagnose someone as to being intoxicated or not. But what I can do is, I smelled ETOH-like odour [referring to an alcohol odour] on the patient's breath and the patient admitted to me to have had ... a twenty-sixer of whatever, right. So if the patient admits to illicit drug use, or if the patient admits to alcohol consumption, or anything like that, I can put that in there, but it has to be completely unbiased. So, and that's the case with *all* of my PCRs ... I have to come up with this very obtuse way of painting the picture for me to go, "in my opinion."

As Julie is explaining how writing the ePCR intertwines with not only biomedical discourse but also legal discourses, Jake interrupts and says that if a patient "forties" on us, meaning refuses to be assessed and/or refuses to go to the hospital, or if there are any extraordinary circumstances, "like if there's an issue on scene with family ... if the family is argumentative ... you're absolutely more diligent with the type of information you put in to justify what you did or didn't do or what the patient said to you." He mentions that, depending on the "odds of something maybe coming back [*laugh*], the greater the liability, the longer the PCR or you put in more pertinent things."

Julie and Jake both explained that the legal environment in which their work takes place can impact it significantly. For example, I noticed during one call where Jake was attending to a patient who was a young woman that he seemed much more cautious when attaching the 12-lead and blood pressure cuff to her. Before this patient, I observed many times where he (and other paramedics) would place some of the electrodes near the breasts of their female patients and do so in a respectful but non-cautious way. This time was different. Jake explained to me that the woman had been "under the influence of stimulants" and "I was just being prudent" for "precautionary purposes" because "you can develop heart issues from it. You can develop ischemic chest pain from that." As a result, he needed to attach electrodes around the patient's chest to ensure that she was not experiencing any heart issues. The work involved in doing this mitigated his worry that the patient would think he was simply "trying to check out her chest." Rather than just placing the electrodes on her chest, Jake asked her "if it was ok for [him] to put it on her or for her to assist herself." Furthermore, and this was a common practice I observed in other paramedics, Jake used the back of his hand to move the breast aside to attach the electrode rather than the front of his hand. His work with the patient, therefore, oriented to the age and gender of the patient and the need to mitigate "risk":

> I try and be respectful, especially with young girls. Old women, they'll [*laugh*] drop their shirt before you even say, "do you mind if I … " They don't care. They don't have no modesty … Legal-wise, you justify why I have to do it, but also, if you have a female partner, I try and do it with her there or have Julie do it … If you do have a partner there, I prefer my female partner to put it on. If there's two guys, well what choice do we have? Like I said legal-wise, people have been charged with sexual assault … and you'll see when we put them on, usually we'll use the back of the hand to push the breast out of the way. Not cupped … With women, Julie and I will use the back of our hand to move the breast out of the way … It's a legal thing. It's a comfort thing. It's a respect thing … It mitigates your risk.

Jake also mentioned that Julie will sometimes turn the mirror and watch what is happening in the back to provide Jake with additional support and to provide another voice if he were to be accused of anything. He characterized this precautionary work as doing additional "little" things to "mitigate liability."

After about 45 minutes of working on the ePCR, Jake exits the ambulance and walks to a little room inside the hospital. I later found out that this was the ePCR room that paramedics use to print off, and sometimes write, their ePCRs. Once it is done, Jake brings the printout to the nursing unit that "we handed the patient off to." Jake quickly returns to the garage and we all load into the ambulance and head off. As we leave the garage, Jake contacts the Dispatch Centre by pressing on his walkie-talkie connected to the CAD and says, "10-48" and someone from the Centre replies, "Unit 208, you're good for 08." "10-48" is coded talk where "10" signifies that the crew has "cleared" from a hospital and "48" refers to which hospital they are clearing from; each hospital has its own number. "208" refers to the unit number of the crew and "08" refers to the station.

We make our way back to the station for what I had originally thought of as "downtime" – time when paramedics are not "working" on the streets. I soon realize that there is very little time to actually be "down."[9] Even if there were extended periods of time between calls (e.g., no call for the remainder of the shift), and paramedics were literally "down" asleep, trying to sleep, "shooting the shit" with other paramedics, or just watching television, I began to view this time as "up" time because paramedics were always gearing towards the "what ifs" of their job – in this context, the possibility of a call or preparing for a call (e.g., teaching work); even during "downtime," paramedics were orienting to the possibilities of their work. For me, this need to be constantly ready made it very difficult to relax during "downtime" and was both mentally and physically draining. Ironically, I was exhilarated by the possibility of the tones going off, which filled me with anticipatory excitement.

"One, Two, Three" – Stretcher Work

We return to the station and I go to the washroom. When I come out, neither Jake, Julie, nor April is in the station. I hear noises coming from the garage so I head out to see what is going on. As I enter the garage, I hear Jake and Julie say in unison, "One, two, three." I begin observing Jake and Julie passionately teach April some of the intricacies of something central to what paramedics do: lifting, loading, and transporting patients on the stretcher. Until now, I have taken what Jake referred to as "stretcher work" for granted, work that he characterized as one of the most important parts of his job because paramedics are always "one lift away from ending their career."[10] April then tells Jake and Julie that she had only practised stretcher work for an hour in her training program, and "it was actually on the flatbed of somebody's truck." Jake replies, "If anything's going to end your career it's going to be this, and they spend an hour on it, *bullshit*." For the next 45 minutes, and with me acting as a mock patient lying on the stretcher with my recorder located between my thighs, I observe and record the complexity of work that goes into what I had previously viewed as the simple and uneventful task of lifting, transporting, and loading patients on a stretcher.

I learned that the height of the paramedic can mediate how far you can actually lift the stretcher; whereas Jake can stand up and the stretcher easily reaches its highest position, both Julie and April are "about an inch out," meaning standing is not enough to lift the stretcher completely to its highest position. Standing there with the

stretcher partly resting on her thick black leather belt, Julie exemplifies to April how she compensates for this as she lets out a big moan
and curls her arms up, while simultaneously going on her tiptoes, and
lifts the stretcher to the necessary position to lock it in place. Julie adds
that lifting is complicated by the height differences between the paramedics doing the lifting: "It doesn't help that he's six one. I'm what,
five six? It makes it a lot harder. So physics is against us. The mechanics is against us." Julie explains to April that she needs to orient to
the imbalance this can create and compensate by lifting the stretcher
a little bit quicker or slower than her partner, depending on whether
she is at the head or the foot. Jake adds that this is further complicated
by tall patients because paramedics will need to sometimes "tilt" their
heads back or to the side to avoid getting "toes in the nose," or to
position the body of the patient to avoid inadvertent "pressure" being
placed on the stretcher, which can activate a "trigger" that can col-
lapse it. This orienting to the "what ifs" of the stretcher needs to be
done artfully; as Jake explains, you "don't do it too much" because
if you do, "that changes your balance, right," which can lead to the
stretcher tipping.

After practising a number of lifts, April starts to rub her right shoulder. Julie takes note of this and tells April that she can work on lifting
the stretcher at a later date. It is not even halfway through the shift yet,
but I need to head home. On my way home, I think about how artful
stretcher work is; paramedics have to take into consideration multiple factors such as the balance of the stretcher, patient characteristics,
partner characteristics, and of course environmental factors, such as
whether there is snow or ice on the ground. They must orient to all of
these complexities by communicating with their partners, listening for
specific noises that the stretcher makes, and modifying and reposition-
ing bodies to avoid a foot in the face and to complete a lift. This work
exemplifies an intricate, contextual, and important part of paramedics'
work, work that I had previously taken for granted as appearing rather
simple on the surface.

Chapter Three

"The Hospital's Going to Complain"

At the Hall

I arrive at the station at around 5:00 pm, about half an hour before the crew I am going to be riding with today is supposed to arrive. I knock on the door to get let in. I am surprised to see Jake, who opens the door and says, "Go away." He turns around and leaves. I stand there awkwardly for about a minute, after which he returns and opens the door and lets out a big laugh. I too let out a big laugh, though I am a bit relieved that Jake came back quickly because I am getting cold; it is the middle of winter and a particularly cold day in Calgary, with temperatures hovering around −15C. After being let in, I walk into the living room and sit down on the couch. Jake walks into the kitchen and begins to make himself some coffee. After his coffee is made, he heads out to the garage. I pick up the backpack that I brought with me and follow him.

As I enter the garage, I notice that Julie is directing puddles of water on the ground with a squeegee to the centre of the floor where a drain is located. Jake walks over to the opposite end of the garage where another squeegee is resting against the wall, picks it up, and joins Julie in pushing the water into the drain. I also notice what looks like a different ambulance from the one I am used to seeing. I would later find out that this ambulance was one of the new standardized units that were being "rolled out" in the province. After about 10 minutes of squeegeeing, Hanna and Dan, paramedics I have ridden with a few times before, arrive. As Dan and Hanna enter the hall, Jake puts the squeegee back in its original place, walks over to the crew, and begins talking and laughing with them. Julie soon joins them. I walk over to the squeegee that

Julie has rested against the wall, pick it up, and begin doing what Julie and Jake were doing.

After a few minutes of chatting, Jake and Julie leave, and Dan and Hanna begin their prepping work, with Hanna inspecting the exterior of the ambulance and Dan in the back. As I enter the truck, I think to myself, "This is different." I take another look around and say to myself again, "Wow, this is different." The ambulance seems much smaller than the previous ambulances I have ridden in. There are still three seats: one airway seat, which I am sitting in, a different style of seat where the bench seat used to be (the seat slides), and the compression seat opposite the rolling seat. I also notice that the cupboards no longer have locks on them. The paramedic has to slide them open. Dan explains that the sliding cupboard is a "good idea" but "it doesn't work" in practice; he cannot open the cupboards with one hand, which "compromises" the ergonomics of the ambulance. I notice that the stretcher looks brand new and is very different from the stretchers I am used to seeing. Whereas the stretchers I have seen before had metallic bars and the cushion was burgundy red, the new stretchers are painted yellow and black, the cushion is black and slightly curved on the edges, and the frame is much bigger and heavier. I also notice that there is no net in the ambulance and I cannot see where the "Christmas tree" that holds the different colour bags is. Lastly, I notice something written on one of the walls. I stand up to read it and realize that I cannot stand up all the way without hitting my head against the ceiling. The writing says, "Demers Ambulances."

As Dan is prepping the ambulance, he turns to me and says, "It goes like stink [fast] but the layout is crap." Hanna, who has now made her way into the unit, interrupts and says the old ambulances were "great" but the "specs" of this new ambulance are designed according to the "Ambulance Services Act." She then explains that the new design is about "safety ... for us." She goes on: "I don't have to stand up any-more although realistically you're gonna have to ... so much of our job you have to get up ... I mean, you can't be sitting down doing compressions. It doesn't work." Dan explains:

> Like the idea of this safety concept is sound, and it's probably good that they're trying to keep us safe but the way that we do our job ... In this unit, there just doesn't seem to be any space to work. Like it's cramped. It seems to be, I don't know if it's narrower or if it's just the stretcher's wider, but there's no room to walk down the sides, and that's already proven to

be, for me anyways, a safety hazard, 'cause there's lots of times where we have to stand up and we're tripping over the stretcher ... Um, there's no room to work. Like there's no place to lay anything out. Like we've got these IV bags and medication bags, we can't, there's nowhere to put them. They've got a little tray under the monitor by the door there on the siding of the back ... that's all your workspace. So there's no place to put anything.

I ask what they do to compensate for the lack of space, and Hanna explains, "Use the patient ... I don't think that's very professional [but] what else are we going to do?" Hanna is referring to how she would have to sometimes rest the electronic Patient Care Record (ePCR), Lifepak, or saline bags on the stretcher, often with the patient on it. I ask them if there is anything else they do to "make more room." Dan mentions how he would often make a makeshift trash can out of "old pink bins" because the waste bin "they've put in at the very bottom of that little stand [is] not very useful." I also noticed during later ride-alongs with this crew that, in order to create or modify the space for working in this ambulance, Dan and Hanna often positioned their bodies to fit within the confines of the unit when in the back with a patient. Whereas the previous ambulance allowed paramedics to sit on the bench seat with their knees perpendicular to the patient and their feet resting at the base of the stretcher with room to spare, the new ambulances did not allow this, especially for taller people. To compensate for this, Dan would angle his knees and feet slightly to the right or left in relation to the base of his body so his knees would not be pushing against the patient and stretcher. From my perspective, observing him while I sat in the airway seat, and in relation to how he used to sit in the older ambulance, this seemed awkward at times for Dan, as the ePCR no longer balanced on his thighs (one thigh was slightly higher than the other) and his positioning in relation to the patient seemed to be out of sorts. Other crews I rode along with also made similar adjustments with their bodies in the new ambulances.

Dan and Hanna both explained how the new structure of the ambulance organizes their work differently compared to the previous ambulances in Calgary, which were based on a design developed with over a decade and a half of input on the uniqueness of working in Calgary – "every series of trucks that [the city] got was a progression; they built on the one previous to make things better." With the new ambulances, Dan explained that how they do something "as simple as starting an IV, which we do all the time," has changed. Previously, starting an IV was typically "defer[red] to the ambulance." Now, according to Dan, it is "going to happen on scene" because "it's so cumbersome to do it back here." While this is not always problematic, Hanna explained how it was going to have a big impact when attending to an "acute patient where you have to decrease your on scene time, right, so you do everything en route," which has now been made more challenging with the newly designed units.

Hospital Relief

About an hour after I arrive at the station, the tones sound. Dan and Hanna, who are now watching TV in the living room, rush to the ambulance, and I follow. Today Hanna is driving and Dan is in the passenger seat, leading the call. Hanna glances at the Computer Aided Dispatch (CAD) mounted between her and Dan on the dashboard of the ambulance and says, "Aw," in a disappointed tone, "Hospital relief." Hospital relief is when a crew relieves another crew who is waiting with a patient at a hospital. The crew at the hospital is usually relieved near the end of their shift and at the beginning of the relieving crews' shift in order to avoid overtime.

I enter the ambulance and we soon depart for the hospital. After about 25 minutes in what seems like a leisurely though bumpy ride in the new ambulance (I also notice that the airway seat is very uncomfortable), we arrive at the hospital at 7:50 pm. The walk to the emergency department (ED) in this hospital is a long one, longer than all of the other hospitals I have been to, about five minutes in total from the garage where the ambulance is parked. Once we arrive at the ED, we walk a bit longer to a well-lit hallway with a few tables placed against the wall and some chairs scattered throughout. Dan leans over and whispers in my ear, "Welcome to the Klein Mile." He is referring to former Premier Ralph Klein, who played an important role in "reforming" the health care system in Alberta beginning in the 1990s.

Halfway down the hallway, two paramedics are waiting with an individual slouched over in a wheelchair. I cannot tell if she is unconscious, but I can see that she is not moving. I look at the patient and notice that she seems to be middle-aged and has darker skin. In my fieldnotes, I write that this individual is a middle-aged aboriginal woman. There is a white bandage around her head, and I can see hints of blood on her face. It is only after the patient attempts to stand up from her wheelchair and nearly falls over that I notice how worn out and beat up she looks; her clothes are dirty and her face looks as though it has been on the receiving end of a fight. In fact, I overhear Hanna ask her if she was in a fight.

I take a seat about five feet away from the wheelchair and observe. I notice that one of the paramedics whom Hanna and Dan would eventually relieve nudges the patient's chair with his foot in a kicking motion. After he nudges the wheelchair, he asks the patient in a loud voice some "orienting" questions like, What day is it? What year and month is it? The patient slurs some words in response that I cannot discern. Hanna quietly says to me that the patient "seems combative" and "intoxicated." I understand what she means by "intoxicated," as indicated by the patient's slurred speech and lethargic demeanour, but it remains unclear to me how she is "combative"; throughout our time with the patient, I observe her remain relatively motionless. However, while she is relatively motionless, as we will see, she is being moved through institutional processes (Diamond, 1992).

Before the paramedics we are replacing leave, Dan and one of them have a quick conversation. Once they finish speaking, the paramedic hands Hanna a printout of his ePCR. I would later find out that the ePCR was also digitally transferred to the ePCR that Hanna was holding. As I sit there observing this exchange between the first crew and Hanna, I see an older patient being "parked" in the hallway where we are located. About 20 minutes after that, an additional paramedic rolls another older patient in to be parked in the hallway. I find this entire unfolding of events – patients parked – unique to my experiences thus far, as there have been only a few times throughout my ride-alongs when I had to wait in the hospital. With that said, as the summer months approached, it seemed as though I would wait more and more.

Once the patient has been transferred to Hanna and Dan, Dan begins to do his own assessment. Hanna walks over to the seat next to me and sits down, which is fortunate because she is able to explain to me what is going on. Once Hanna sits down, and as I take my recorder out, Dan begins his assessment with a blood "poke" to measure the patient's blood sugar level. He then asks the patient a lot of questions: "Have you been drinking today?" "Where does it hurt?" "Are you pregnant?" "Hep C, HIV, anything like that?" These questions are followed by other "orienting" questions, according to Hanna, such as, "What's the date? Your name? What happened?"

As Hanna and I are talking, I hear the patient and Dan interacting in the background. "Sit up," Dan says to the patient, and the patient asks, "What?" Dan replies in a mocking tone, "What?" Dan then states, "What's going on? Where do you hurt?" I do not discern a response from the patient, though it became clear when Dan spoke to me later about writing the ePCR that this non-response was entered into the ePCR as an indication of the level of the patient's alertness. Hanna explains to me that, based on the patient's responses (and non-responses), Dan has decided to board her because she is an "unreliable patient" who cannot answer any of the previous questions and is thus "altered if you will." Referencing the C-Spine protocol (see figure 3.1), Hanna explains to me why they are about to place the patient on a board, secure her to it, and restrict her ability to move her neck.

> She has had trauma. We don't know how she got that but there's obviously some sort of trauma. Did she fall? I don't know. Was she punched in the head? I don't know. She has alcohol on board ... Those are all signs for us to put her on a backboard because she could have some sort of head injury.

Soon after Dan's assessment, Dan, with Hanna's assistance, moves a stretcher near us that already has a board placed on it next to the patient and gently helps her on. To secure the patient, they tighten some straps that intermesh with the board around the patient's body. Once strapped in, the patient asks for a blanket and says, "I'm cold." Dan tells her that he will get her a blanket shortly but that he needs to first start an IV. Hanna hands Dan a needle from the red bag. Before Dan inserts the IV, he tells the patient in a loud, stern, and stringent voice, "Don't move," and says this at least two more times before he "pokes" the patient. As Dan is getting ready to insert the needle, the patient says that she wants to be unstrapped.

Dan says, "One, two, three," and, as he quickly and elegantly inserts the needle into the patient's right arm, he simultaneously says, "Ouch, ouch, ouch." He later explained to me that he does this for two reasons: 1) to prepare the patient for the anticipated pain of the needle being inserted, and 2) in the process of preparing the patient for the pain, it has been his experience that the patient is less likely to pull away as the needle is being inserted. After the needle has been inserted, tape is placed on the needle, pulled around it, and stuck to the skin to secure it in place. Dan then asks the patient some questions, including "Where do you stay?" "Do you have a home?" The patient, who seems to be

3.1 The C-Spine protocol

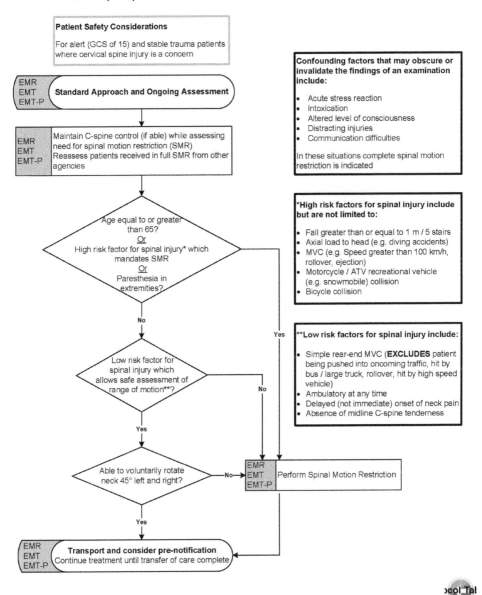

Patient Safety Considerations

For alert (GCS of 15) and stable trauma patients where cervical spine injury is a concern

EMR / EMT / EMT-P — **Standard Approach and Ongoing Assessment**

EMR / EMT / EMT-P — Maintain C-spine control (if able) while assessing need for spinal motion restriction (SMR) Reassess patients received in full SMR from other agencies

Age equal to or greater than 65? **Or** High risk factor for spinal injury* which mandates SMR **Or** Paresthesia in extremities?

Low risk factor for spinal injury which allows safe assessment of range of motion**?

Able to voluntarily rotate neck 45° left and right?

EMR / EMT / EMT-P — Perform Spinal Motion Restriction

EMR / EMT / EMT-P — **Transport and consider pre-notification** Continue treatment until transfer of care complete

Confounding factors that may obscure or invalidate the findings of an examination include:

- Acute stress reaction
- Intoxication
- Altered level of consciousness
- Distracting injuries
- Communication difficulties

In these situations complete spinal motion restriction is indicated

*High risk factors for spinal injury include but are not limited to:

- Fall greater than or equal to 1 m / 5 stairs
- Axial load to head (e.g. diving accidents)
- MVC (e.g. Speed greater than 100 km/h, rollover, ejection)
- Motorcycle / ATV recreational vehicle (e.g. snowmobile) collision
- Bicycle collision

**Low risk factors for spinal injury include:

- Simple rear-end MVC (**EXCLUDES** patient being pushed into oncoming traffic, hit by bus / large truck, rollover, hit by high speed vehicle)
- Ambulatory at any time
- Delayed (not immediate) onset of neck pain
- Absence of midline C-spine tenderness

December 1, 2010   C-Spine Assessment Protocol

Source: © 2014 Alberta Health Services. See Acknowledgments for further attribution and disclaimer (Alberta Health Services 2010a).

3.2 C-Spine Experience

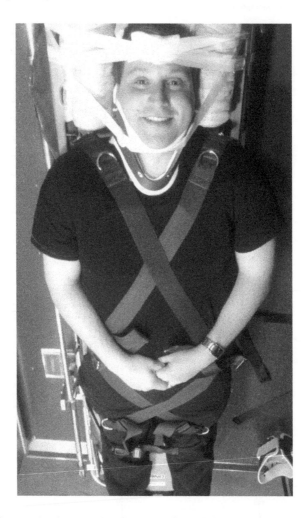

On a later ride-along with Jake and Julie, while waiting in the ambulance at one of the hospitals, Julie suggested that I try the C-Spine. I was curious, so I agreed. Julie placed the brace around my neck, almost completely immobilizing it, and I soon felt what I could only describe as an almost complete loss of control. It was the slight ability to move my neck that reminded me that I was still in control of trying out this intervention. After the brace was secured, I lay down, as instructed by Julie, on the stretcher, which already had the C-Spine board placed on top of it. It was uncomfortable to say the least, as if I had lain down on a hard floor. Julie and Jake soon began to strap me in, which I was fine with. I could still move my head and to a certain extent my legs. Then they began to tighten the straps. All of a sudden, one of the paramedics (I could no longer move my head so I could not see who) held my head in place and the other began placing tape around it and connecting it to the stretcher. I became extremely anxious, though I put on a front and remained calm and cool. Julie and Jake then explained to me that, if necessary, they could strap my hands down. After lying there for a few seconds, I tried to move. I could not. "Don't do that again," I remember thinking to myself, as I became even more anxious about not being able to move. This is when it hit me. I had no control. Soon after, Julie took a picture of me with her cellphone. The slight smile in the picture is an inauthentic one; at this point, I had lost any feelings of control, and feelings of claustrophobia were taking over. Before they let me out, Jake tilted me over onto my side and explained to me that, if necessary, they could do a little bit of "street medicine." He then began to kick the bottom of the C-Spine with his steel-toed boots, which reverberated throughout my entire body.

talking more clearly now, says that she lives in a shelter and that she would like bus tickets to go home. Dan then asks Hanna if they should "draw some [medication] up." Hanna replies, "You've got the nukes," referring to the drugs they carry in the pouch on their person. She then hands Dan another needle from the red bag. Dan takes the needle and inserts it into a small vial. He slowly pulls the lever attached to the needle to capture some of the liquid. Dan tells the patient that the medicine will "help you relax." "I'll give her 2.5," Dan says to Hanna. As Dan administers the drug by putting the needle into a slot in the IV, I notice Hanna looking through the protocol book. The entire process of drawing the drugs and administering them takes about a minute. Although I cannot discern what page(s) she is looking at, there is a "combative behaviour protocol" in the book, which states, among other things, that patients should be given "2.5 mg or 5.0 mg" of "Midazolam," with the lower dosage being given to patients who are over the age of 65 or have a "smaller body mass" (AHS, 2010a). When Dan finishes administering the drug, he says in a loud voice, "2.5," which is followed by a quick tap by Hanna on the ePCR.

Once the drug has been administered, Dan tells the patient, "Do not move your arm. I'll tie you down." As Dan begins walking towards the triage desk, Hanna says that he is "updating" the nurse. I ask Hanna to explain what she means by "updating" the nurse and she says, "So he went to triage to update them that we were going to be doing a new treatment. As the patient came in in a wheelchair and we're obviously putting her on a board, which immediately bumps her up in, 'cause they don't like to keep people on a backboard too long."

I have noticed that, between these sequences of events, Hanna is tapping on the ePCR. When Dan leaves to update the nurse, I ask her why she is doing this. She explains, "I was documenting the drug that we gave. The route that we gave it, which was through the IV. And the amount that we gave her." She goes on:

> HANNA: I'm going to put in these vitals, so I just tap on vital signs and add. So this is the time, so I enter the time. The heart rate is 100. Tap. I would guess she's breathing at about [*inaudible*] per minute. Blood pressure, just tap that in. That's another screen. Stats are 87. This is her um, how alert she is. So her eyes are open spontaneously. I'm going to call her confused because she couldn't answer all those orientation questions.
>
> M: You're giving her a GCS [Glasgow Coma Scale] of 14.[1]
>
> HANNA: Yeah. So, and then her motor response, so she obeys commands. So if we tell her to stand up, she can do it. That kind of stuff. And then enter.

As our conversation continues, she talks about the "treatment" section of the ePCR. With the tap of a button, Hanna "logs" in Dan's treatments, which consists of entering in the drug "that we gave" and recording how it was given. While continuing to enter information, Hanna explains, "Dan put the IV in the right forearm. It was a successful attempt. He tried one time using a size 18 needle." She says that the patient's "medical status" has not changed based on the treatments they did. She also says that there were no "complications. Save.

And then we did spinal motion restrictions. So we did c-collar spine board blanket roll straps."

Upon returning to the patient's side, Dan takes what looks like a thick rope and begins to tie the patient's arms to the side rails of the stretcher. Looking over Hanna's shoulder with the ePCR placed open on her lap, I notice that she records in the "treatment" section that Dan did restraints. As Dan is doing the restraints, a person wearing a uniform that says "security" on it comes to finish the restraints that Dan has started. As the security officer is restraining the patient, I hear the patient say in her clearest yet still slurring words, "I'm not comfortable," which is soon followed by "Why are you doing this to me?" After the security officer finishes his work of restraining, he walks over to Dan and asks for his name and badge number. While this is happening, I hear the patient say, "I don't need to be in here." Dan asks Hanna if he should give the patient another "2.5."[2] Hanna responds in the affirmative and a similar process of drawing the liquid from the vial ensues. After the drugs are administered, the patient becomes quiet.

Soon after "updating" the triage nurse, at around 8:57 pm, the paramedics begin the process of transferring the patient to the hospital; a bed must have become available. As Hanna is rolling the patient to one of the units on the ward, as instructed by the triage nurse to Dan, I notice that the patient looks unconscious; she is not saying anything, nor is she moving. Once we arrive at the unit, the nurse there, to whom Dan passes on information, asks, "Why is she boarded?" Dan replies, "Bear with me, we're the fourth crew to have her." Dan goes on to account for his decision to board the patient. He explains that, based on the notes he received in the ePCR and the verbal exchange with the previous crew, he thought it was the correct and prudent course of action; he says that he did not know how the patient fell and if she hit her head or hurt her neck (the patient was not able to answer these questions). In the middle of Dan's conversation with the nurse, a doctor arrives, stands behind the nurse, folds his arms across his chest, and appears to listen to their interchange. Dan explains to the nurse why he did what he did, and the nurse comments that she saw the first crew bring the patient in and thought they were "snarky." This exchange lasts about four minutes. After Dan's explanation to the nurse, the patient is placed in the space that has been allocated to her in the ED.

I follow Hanna out to the garage and into the back of the ambulance. Dan joins us and says in a serious tone, "The hospital's going to complain."

DAN: It turns out, did you get the run-down on our patient, like what happened?

M: Not really.

DAN: From what it shows on the [ePCR] report that we got, it was that she had a fall, uh, an unwitnessed fall, which is vital information. So the fall was unwitnessed, so we don't really know 100 per cent if it was a fall. We just know that she was bleeding ... from one head wound in an alley. She's got alcohol on board and she's uh cannot recall the events. So that right there, criteria for us to really kind of take this situation rather seriously because we don't know what happened to her and um, is she altered from a head injury or is she just altered from the alcohol? That's impossible for us to determine. So that's kind of why we took the measures that we did um, because now she needs to be worked up ... It's easy to pass somebody off as being drunk. She's admitted to drinking. She smells like alcohol. She's probably drunk. But it's impossible for us to make that determination.

M: I noticed with your interchange with the nurse that you kind of had to justify why she was placed into the C-Spine.

DAN: Yes. This nurse apparently was at the triage desk when this patient came in ... So this patient was brought in by another crew. She was brought in walking. Um [*sigh*], now again, I was not at the scene, I cannot explain to you why, the crew that brought her in chose to bring her in like that. I can't explain to you their rationale but even, the triage nurse seemed to kind of agree with me, so, she said, "Well this patient was brought in on a wheelchair. How come she's on a spine board now?" And so basically I had to explain to her why I felt it was necessary for her to be placed on a spine board and to be spinal immobilized, right, 'cause we're concerned about obviously spinal cord injuries. If you ask me, she should have been brought to the hospital packaged like that, right. Um, it's detrimental to the patient, right, if they're not, right, again because we do not know the extent of her injuries and it's impossible to know the extent of her injuries without an X-ray, CT scan, you know MRI if necessary. She needs to be assessed by a doctor. I can pretty much guarantee you she's not coming off of that board until there's at least X-rays.

On another ride-along, Julie and Jake talked about how they "package" their patients in certain ways; however, this conversation was in a different context. Julie explained, for instance, that most patients they transport to hospital "probably don't need IVs"; however, paramedics do IVs "to be nice" and "it's partly selling our patient." Jake goes on:

> Part of playing the game here … A happy nurse can be a friend to you [*laugh*]. That's why I don't mind changing the patient if we have time – put him into a gown. They [hospital staff] appreciate it. And most of the time they'll say thank you … It saves them time. So there's times you do things for them to help the flow of the system work, other times, like, "No, this is inappropriate this time."

Part of what I observed on this call was how paramedics orient to different social characteristics of their patients.[3] Connecting to the "prejudging work" discussed in chapter 2, one of the things I found interesting about this call was how Hanna "guess[ed] that she's probably a regular drinker," which, according to her, impacted the course of treatment Dan provided. She explained that if the patient is a regular drinker, it "is more likely she could have a head bleed. It just thins out the blood." I asked Hanna to explain why she thought the patient was a regular drinker. She replied, "She's uh, she's um, she's poor hygiene, she stays at the Drop In Centre, and just from, not that everybody who has those things is a drinker, but just from experience with this kind of clientele, that I can guess. Whether that's true or not, I don't know … so we err on the side of caution and put her on the board." This understanding of the patient was central to why, as Hanna explained, they decided to give the patient some sedation drugs; not only was the patient uncomfortable, according to Hanna, but "we anticipated she might be combative trying to put her on the board. She wasn't, which was good." Furthermore, they started an IV to give the patient some fluids because "she might be malnourished. Again with that clientele, often they're not well nourished."

What I found interesting when reflecting on this call was how this prejudgment work was non-existent, perhaps necessarily so, when Dan explained to the nurse why he decided to board the patient; much of the reasoning behind his decision disappeared or was subsumed into his explanation of what he did as being a "prudent course of action." This explanation also connects, as we saw with Julie's account in chapter 2 of why she did not board her Motor Vehicle Collision (MVC) patient, to the C-Spine protocol that states that "complete spinal motion restriction is indicated" if the patient is "intoxicated," has an "altered level of consciousness," and has "communication difficulties" (AHS, 2010a, p. 102). Perhaps more relevant is how the paramedic's work orients and responds to the context, yet this contingency work disappears in the writing of the ePCR, perhaps necessarily so for different purposes; we see that the "Cole's Notes" version of what happened (see chapter 2), as told by the paramedic to the triage nurse and unit nurse, is to expedite the transfer of the patient, whereas the institutional account, as recorded in the ePCR, is to create a common standard of measurability for statistical and accountability purposes.

A Lack of Sympathy?

Part of what also intrigued me about this observation was how these paramedics interacted with this patient, an interaction that I felt demonstrated a lack of sympathy towards the patient. Such an interaction was not characteristic of the majority of my observations; the paramedics I observed during my ride-alongs appeared, for the most part, very understanding and sympathetic towards their patients, intoxicated or not. However, the few observations where I observed a lack of sympathy primarily occurred when the patient was intoxicated.

As I reflected on this observation, I remembered a conversation with one paramedic, Sam, who spoke specifically about "sympathy," or the lack thereof, on the front lines of emergency health services. He discussed how the "job changes you" so that, over time, he developed a lack of sympathy and became "very cynical" towards a specific group of "clientele," primarily intoxicated individuals and/or patients from a particular ethnic background.[4] With some hesitation in his voice, combined with what appeared to be a bit of embarrassment or an apologetic tone that was only partially displaced by his desire to tell me about a topic of utmost importance to him, he explained the following:

> This job has forced me to lose a lot of respect, for example, with Natives. I'm very intolerable [intolerant] of them now, because you see how so many, and I realize that they're not all like this, but you see how so many of them take advantage ... and you are going out there to deal with them with the same things all the time, and they're always drunk ... and when you see them abuse the system ... and you get so frustrated with stuff

like that, and you become very cynical of lots of different things ... Like here's a good example of something that we'll see on a regular basis is, pancreatitis is not all the time, but it is a lot of the time it is caused by drinking, alcoholics, they get pancreatitis, and it's very painful, you get nauseous with it ... and they know what happens when they drink. They will go out and they'll drink, and they'll get drunk, and then they'll develop pancreatitis, and then they call me, and now all of the sudden it's my problem, and now I have to give them pain medication, and now I have to take them to the hospital ... Half the time ... Most [of] the time because they're alcoholics they don't pay the fucking ambulance bill, so the ambulance bill never gets paid, it incurs costs to the medical system, and now I have to be sympathetic to your abdominal pain and nausea that you've brought on yourself when you know that you shouldn't be doing this? You tell me why I should feel sympathy for you? I don't feel the least bit sympathetic for you ... and you see this stuff repeatedly, you see it repeatedly, and it jades you; you get frustrated, and you get pissed off, and you ... When you see what human beings do to each other, and you see what they do to themselves, and how they treat other people, how they treat animals, how they treat property, and it's just such a waste of human life, that's where your jaded comes from, right? Right there you're like, "Oh, we're going here again," you know, and you recognize addresses. Tones will go off, you'll walk out to the CAD, "Oh, we're going to so-and-so's house again," you know exactly who it is, you know where they live, and you know what you're going for, and unfortunately, hopefully those people aren't going to cry wolf and be actually in a position where now they actually need you, but they've cried wolf so many times that the rest of us are just like whatever, you know? And people that don't see it ... look at us and think like you're an asshole ... and we joke about it; we sit around and we joke about it with each other, because a large majority of us experience that and/or feel that way, and it's a common thing.

Sam's talk consisted of two interrelated themes where he viewed aboriginal and intoxicated patients as abusing the system. His talk was organized by discourses of individual/personal culpability (self-responsibilizing discourses) and discourses of the "right" or deserving patients. In addition to discussing how certain patients "take advantage" of the system, which potentially has consequences for his well-being as a front-line worker – "Every time we go lights and sirens, we put ourselves and everyone else in jeopardy" – he mentioned how his work orients to and is mediated by this demographic of "clientele" where, according to his partner Inese, "aggressiveness comes in a little bit ... Your anger comes out a little bit ... [*exemplifying how she might speak to the patient*] 'OK, get up. This is inappropriate. You can't be lying here.'"

In the course of their work, paramedics come face-to-face with many people who are suffering in society. Such individuals are overrepresented in specific social categories because of broad and pervasive social determinants that structure individual experiences of and responses to health and illness in society. The work of paramedics described here is interesting because it tells us how paramedics orient to their patients' different social categories and sheds some light on how society is put together in ways that reproduce these experiences for paramedics. We can learn from the work processes of paramedics and how they engage with larger-scale issues of health and inequality.

Furthermore, Sam's talk draws attention to the stresses experienced by front-line health workers. Paramedics and other front-line workers, for example, experience exceptionally high rates of "burnout" and other negative outcomes that are invariably connected to their work setting. Sam's talk reminded me of the work of Paul Farmer (1996), who discusses how social forces become "embodied as individual experience" (p. 262). He uses the term "structural violence" to draw attention to how social, political, economic, and historical forces are central to people's experiences of illness and likelihood of becoming ill. While this term is useful to better understand why individuals become sick, I suggest that it is insightful in light of Sam's talk above because it draws attention to how social structures organize the suffering individuals' experience, including front-line health care workers; the stress paramedics and other front-line health care workers experience is inseparable from and organized by their work settings and broader social forces. While social forces structure the types of patients Sam interfaces with on a daily basis, the same social forces structure the "violence" he experiences in his work setting; we cannot address the latter without addressing the former. Andrea Campbell (2013) sheds light on this when she writes about workers in long-term residential care (LTRC) settings:

> Focusing on individual factors connected to health and safety further perpetuates the notion that the health and safety issues of workers are not subject to institutional and societal action. It also conceals the way health

and safety concerns are inseparable from the conditions and relations that structure the organization of their LTRC work ... (p. 95)

There is a need to ground such conversations about "burnout" and other forms of "violence" in the actual work settings of paramedics and their experiences in those work settings in order to begin to address the broader issues that organize such experiences.

Downtime – Coffee

About 45 minutes after we arrive in the garage of the hospital, and after Dan has finished writing his ePCR, we leave. On the way to the station, we stop for a cup of coffee. While we are walking into the coffee shop, someone waiting in line at the drive-thru rolls down her window, offers Hanna a 20-dollar bill, and expresses her gratitude for the services paramedics do. Hanna thanks the individual but explains to her that paramedics are not allowed to accept money from the public. We then have a quick laugh and walk into the coffee shop, place our order, and take a seat.

As we sit at the coffee shop chatting, suddenly, and before the coffee even arrives, the paramedics get up and walk towards the ambulance parked in the parking lot. Apparently we have a call. We enter the ambulance and Dan informs me that the call has been cancelled. Hanna goes back into the coffee shop and grabs the coffees, and we head back to the hall. It was only after I had children that I began to understand the work that goes into what I had just observed. For example, in learning how to discern the subtle noises that come from the room of newborn babies (we had twins), my partner and I would often try to guess which child it was who was crying; we soon became experts in not only hearing very quiet noises coming from the room, but also in determining who in fact was crying. This skill became most apparent when we had friends over for dinner. After our children were asleep (so we thought or, more accurately, hoped) and while everyone else was chatting loudly, my partner and I would quickly make eye contact and were activated by these subtle noises, often resulting in some negotiating of whose turn it was to tend to our children. I think of this work as similar to Dan and Hanna orienting towards specific and skilfully heard information voiced over their radios from the Dispatch Centre; they oriented to the information that I could not hear and reacted to it.

I began to understand this work as the constant vigilance that is central to what paramedics do.

Once we arrive at the station, I walk to the living room, sit down, and begin watching TV. Dan walks over to the refrigerator, pulls a container from it, places it in the microwave, and presses a few buttons. As he is standing at the microwave, Hanna takes a seat in the armchair. After Dan has waited about two minutes by the microwave, a beep goes off and he grabs his dinner, brings it over to where Hanna and I are seated, and takes a seat in the other chair. We sit there watching television for some time. After about two hours, I stand up and get ready to leave. I thank Dan and Hanna for letting me observe them today and let them know I will see them in a couple of weeks.

"I've Been Burned Several Times"

While driving home, I reflected on the observations I had of the hospital relief. I wondered why a bed became available soon after the patient was placed on the C-Spine board, after she had been parked for some time. In addition, I thought about Dan's comment that the "hospital's going to complain" and wondered why. While I did not have the opportunity to speak with the paramedics who had treated the patient before us, Hanna, Dan, and the nurse suggested that "professional codes and standards" had not been followed by the previous crews; if the work of the previous paramedics was "*not* organized by or oriented to professional codes and [professional] standards, what *is* its organizing principle or focus?" (Rankin & Campbell, 2006, p. 49). This observation activated for me a need to reflect on the socially structured settings that, likely unintentionally, subverted some of the standards of paramedics' profession (p. 49). I thought about the different work orientations of these front-line workers and how they interconnect in some way with resource allocation geared towards garnering "efficiencies" in the health sector and, connected to this, the discourse of putting the "right" patient in the "right" place at the "right" time; both ideas are central to reform practices in the province.

For example, after the patient was transferred to the hospital, Hanna explained that activating the C-Spine protocol and placing the patient on the board, combined with Dan walking to the triage nurse and making her aware of their new treatment, "immediately bumps her [the patient] up in ... 'cause they don't like to keep people on a backboard too long."[5] Hanna's socially organized language – "bumps her up" – points to institutional criteria that determine urgency of treatment in emergency departments. I began to think about how placing the patient on the board was a significantly different treatment from that provided by the crews who treated the patient before we arrived for relief; when we first met the patient, she was slouched over in a wheelchair, which further contrasted with the first crew's attempt, according to Dan, to "download" her into the waiting room with other walk-in patients. While Dan described this relief as an "anomaly" because they do not typically "take over and do a fully different treatment plan," based on what I observed and heard this day, I began to think about how this observation shed light on some of the different work strategies paramedics have available to them at the EMS-ED interface that are geared towards facilitating paramedics in getting back out on the streets.

The process of downloading a patient into the waiting room where she waits by herself until a hospital bed becomes available is one work strategy available to paramedics geared towards increasing "efficiency" in EMS. The decision to download a patient is ultimately up to the triage nurse and is based on information that the nurse gathers from the paramedic, patient, and/or medical devices. The information garnered interfaces with "guidelines" that outline specific "inclusion" and "exclusion" criteria that have to be met in order for a patient to be downloaded into the waiting room. Triage nurse Pam explained:

> So, they also brought out criteria for EMS patients going to the waiting room, so there was a list. It was kind of like a protocol that we had to follow; if this patient had this, this, and this, they can go to the waiting room, but if they had this, this, and this, then they can't go to the waiting room for half an hour. Like so if they were given meds, for example, they couldn't go in the waiting room for obvious reasons, right? Like you can't give a patient morphine and put them in the waiting room, right. So, that was another thing was to decrease wait times for EMS was if they had this stuff, they were stable, they could go to the waiting room. I mean it's always been like that, but because there was always tension[6] they had to actually come up with a list.

This work strategy of the nurse contrasts with other strategies available to paramedics, either past or present, geared towards getting them back out on the streets, including waiting with the patient in the hospital hallway until a bed becomes available, a paramedic unit "doubling up" with another paramedic unit, or paramedic units transferring the care of their patient to a "transfer of care paramedic." For example, some of the paramedics I observed spoke about Transfer of Care Paramedics (TOCPs) that are currently used to transfer patients between hospitals in Calgary. As I understood it, in the past, TOCPs were also used to lessen the number of paramedics parked in the hospitals by allowing street paramedics to transfer the care of their patient to a TOCP. Essentially, Transfer of Care Paramedics facilitated street paramedics in getting back out on the streets and therefore limited the amount of waiting that street paramedics did in the ED. According to Julie, this program was cancelled because it was a "huge failure"; TOCPs "worked hard at not working." Julie explained that when she read newspaper articles about TOCPs and how they were being used to reduce wait times, it disappointed her so much that "I could feel my blood pressure go up ... That's pure bullshit! That's not the way it works. That's the way it works on paper."

Another strategy that paramedics have available to them is a policy whereby, if there are multiple paramedic units waiting in the ED, one unit is supposed to double up or transfer the care of their patient to another paramedic unit that is waiting; one paramedic unit would therefore have two patients and the other paramedic unit would be "clear" to go back on the streets. Julie explained that this policy is "supposed to be that way all the time. Our bosses really don't enforce it." Rather than this policy being enforced "all the time" by her "bosses," Julie explained that paramedics activate it at their discretion.[7] She explained, "Some crews are really, really good at saying, 'Hey, how long have you been here? Oh jeez Mike you guys have been here for three hours. Go print off your PCR and give me your patient. Give me your report and give me your patient.'"

Nevertheless, the work of Dan and Hanna, and the previous crews that tended to this patient, in part organized the responses of the nurse and doctor when, for example, the nurse mentioned to Dan that the first crew was "snarky" to her, and when the doctor listened intently to Dan as he said to the nurse, "Just bear with me," while Dan accounted for and justified his treatment decisions. I began to see the talk between the nurse and Dan, and the observations of the doctor, as a moment of tension that carried social organization; I wondered if these observations connected to what some of the paramedics and nurses I spoke with referred to as paramedics "playing" up or down their patients. Pam explained that because paramedics "know the [download] criteria," they will sometimes "downplay things and tell you things so that they, because they know the criteria so they'll say those things so they can go to the waiting room, but then like an hour later the patient comes up and it's a totally different story and you're like, what?" Furthermore, on a later ride-along, as Julie and I waited in a hospital garage for Jake to finish writing his ePCR, Julie spoke to me about a practice that she viewed with much disdain where paramedics present their patient to the triage nurse as sicker (play up) or healthier (play down) than the patient really is. Another paramedic, Dave, who has nearly 20 years of EMS experience, explained it as follows:

> DAVE: Then there's other [nurses] that just, you know for whatever reason don't like us … I understand why some nurses don't trust medics because some guys will come in and misrepresent what's wrong with the patient so they can get a bed or in order to throw them in the waiting room. And uh, a triage nurse only has to get burned once or twice for that then she, basically they just blanket us all.
>
> M: So when you say misrepresent, how do you do that?
>
> DAVE: They won't tell the whole story or they'll make the patient out as if there's really not that much wrong with them.

Similarly, even though Meg (triage nurse) said that she's been "burned several times," she described being burned as a relatively rare experience.[8] Nevertheless, she spoke about how this practice creates tension between paramedics and nurses and is therefore "distressing" because some nurses "can't trust some of the medics [because] of what they've said and what they do or what they haven't done for a patient." Being burned, or the prospect of being burned, is part of this nurse's work orientation; she orients to the possibility that paramedics do not like to be "parked" with their patients and therefore may deploy work strategies to get out of the hospital faster, sometimes manipulating institutional policies to achieve the goal of increasing "efficiency."

Keeping the institution in view (McCoy, 2006), I examined my observation of the relief shift and the talk about paramedics playing patients up or down as work that is socially organized by the institutional settings in which that work occurs. I thought about how the problematic work practices described above are mediated, albeit broadly, by socially organized practices connected to reform and restructuring practices that categorize patients and allocate hospital spaces (e.g., CTAS) and/or criteria for transferring patients to

the waiting room in order to utilize health care resources more efficiently. I began to think that such reform practices locate nurses and
paramedics in both complementary and, as exemplified in my observations of the relief shift, divergent ways in terms of how their work
is organized and targeted as possible solutions to health care crises.

As mentioned above, paramedics seemed to detest being parked in
the hospital – an experience described by some as "shift killers" and
"suck[ing] the life" out of them – and hence orient to their mandate of
working on the streets. "Good" triage nurses, according to some paramedics, are those who "shuffle" patients around and "just bend over
backwards to get us outta here." On one call, for example, I observed
Julie and Jake parked in the ED hallway with an incontinent patient
even though, according to Julie, beds were open. After the patient was
transferred to the ED, I asked Julie what the difference was between a
good and a bad triage nurse and she explained that a good triage nurse
would not "put us in the hall with a bunch of empty beds ... I kind of
understand what she wanted. She said he was incontinent feces, so she
put him in a negative pressure room so that the stink wouldn't bug everyone else, right. That being said, that's not my problem. Send an NA
[nursing aide] out and wipe his ass, get rid of the poop smell."

Similarly, nurses, like paramedics, orient to their mandate of treating patients, but their mandate is oriented towards the ED, not "the
streets." This mandate interfaces with another and more divergent
mandate in relation to paramedics; triage nurses are also tasked with
managing the resources in the ED in terms of hospital beds, resources
that paramedics deeply rely on to get back out on the streets. Hence
the triage nurses I spoke with oriented to this need to allocate hospital
resources and the possibility of a "big heart attack" (Meg) coming in at
any time or a patient "quickly turn[ing]" (Pam). While beds might be
open in the emergency department – one nurse explained that paramedics sometimes "actually go and walk around ... in the department
and they would say to, you know, they'd look around for an empty bed
and then they'd come back and say well, you know such and such bed
is clean ... Which created more tension ..." – Pam described how she
looks to match the "right" patient to the "right" type of bed that reflects
the needs of the patient. For example, there are monitored and non-
monitored beds, with some patients, like those experiencing chest pain
and breathing difficulties, more in need of a monitored bed than others.
In addition to having more technologies, like a cardiac monitor, these
beds are usually staffed by more "senior nurses" because they "have

more experience to be able to recognize when somebody's sort of getting worse" (Pam). This is in contrast to "an older [patient] that doesn't get around very much then they can't go to that area, so they wait for a non-monitor bed" (Meg).

Furthermore, both of the nurses I spoke to explained that they sometimes make space while dually providing the best care possible by using paramedics in ways that address the realities of the fact that "beds are a premium." Pam explained,

Well, for example the other night we had four patients that were like a CTAS 2 [sick patients who need to be admitted soon], right, and two of them were in the waiting room and two of them were EMS. So, a lot of the times, again, we're always sort of more concerned about the patients in the waiting room; we are responsible for them and at any time we can bring them in and check on them, but we're always a little bit more comfortable when a CTAS patient is with EMS. So, a lot of the times if they come in at the same time we'll put the patient in the waiting room that's a CTAS 2 in. Now, that's not everybody but that's what I do … like the other night when I know that there's beds coming up then I'll usually put the waiting room CTAS 2 in first before the paramedics.

Similarly, Meg explained:

You know, maybe I have someone out in the waiting room, and for me some of that priority is that person out in the waiting room has no one looking after them, whereas the paramedics, the patient on the stretcher has a set of paramedics looking after them and I think that's more important that they have that professional, that this patient in the waiting room has no professional other than us and if it's really busy you don't have the time to be doing, looking, you know, always looking after this person to make sure they're OK until you get them in.

In contrast, Pam explained, "a lot of nurses will as soon as they see paramedics they want to get them back on the street so they'll put them [the paramedics' patients] in first … " Meg voiced similar sentiments as she explained that some nurses put patients in inappropriate beds – "There are some differences in how they triage at the two [hospitals she works at]. I have to admit that you know sometimes they will put people into spots at [her current hospital] that I would go like holy crap I wouldn't put them there, but they're saying well, you know, that's a bed, to facilitate medics getting out on the streets." Such work strategies exemplify how nurses are under pressure to put the right patient in the right place at the right time based on institutional expectations. Both of the nurses I spoke to explained that some nurses place patients in inappropriate beds in order to facilitate more efficient use of EMS resources.

Triage nurses' work is geared to the non-standard context in which it occurs. This work orientation is sometimes in tension with the managerial agenda, which is aligned with paramedics' own preferences, of getting pre-hospital emergency workers out of the hospital and back on the streets as quickly as possible. Here, having/parking paramedics in the hospital is conceptualized institutionally as an "inefficient" use of resources. Furthermore, the descriptions and work orientations described above draw attention to the blurry institutional line of jurisdictional accountability that paramedics and their patients teeter on, on a daily basis; while paramedics and their patient might physically be in the hospital, they are only officially in the hospital once the textual practice of transferring the patient is completed.

The socially organized work practice of getting patients in and paramedics out of the hospital faster but potentially not having beds available when they are needed for unexpected emergencies is in tension with the mandate of triage nurses to provide the best quality of care to their patients and the institutional discourse of putting the right patient in the right place at the right time. In other words, work orientations are being lined up with reform mandates that are "articulated with and *disciplined by* a managerial calculus of resources and priorities" (Clarke & Newman, 1997, p. 76). Furthermore, this social organization can be seen as conflicting with other discourses related to reform practices, specifically the discourse that "we are one. One team. One Board. One plan for the delivery of health care in Alberta."[9] In fact, Meg explained, a paramedic's "playing" the patient up or down is "distressing" because "you want to be able to rely on that team member, because he's really part of the team, or she, and sometimes you can't because of that."

Such work processes as explicated here can result in hidden consequences from well-intentioned reform geared towards getting paramedics out of the hospital faster and putting the "right" patient in the "right" place at the "right" time, and thus limiting the amount of "waste." These consequences were exemplified when Dan said that "the hospital's going to complain," when the nurses spoke about "distress" associated with getting paramedics out of the ED and their changing mandate, and when paramedics distinguished between what constitutes a "good" and "bad" nurse and how paramedics sometimes might "play" their patients up or down in order to leave the hospital quicker. I also began to think that this social organization of admitting and resource allocation in the emergency department permeates the pre-hospital setting and connects, at least in part, to what constitutes a "good" and "shit" (Palmer, 1983a, p. 167) call. Within this social organization, there are institutional processes at work that may contribute to drawing the contours of what counts as an emergency, which organizes the doings of front-line workers with unseen and unforeseen consequences.

Chapter Four

"That Was a Gooder"

"Cold Cocked"

I arrive at the station at 5:30 am. As I get out of my car, an ambulance drives up to the station and opens the garage door. I give the crew a quick wave as I run in front of them and enter the garage. Before the ambulance is fully parked, I walk through the garage and through the side door that leads into the living room and kitchen area. As I enter, I see Jake and Julie eating breakfast; Julie is eating some fruit and yogurt and Jake is eating a breakfast sandwich from Tim Hortons. Both are also holding extra large coffees from Tim Hortons. I say good morning and Jake says that there is a coffee for me in the kitchen. I head over to the kitchen and pick up my coffee. As I return to the television area, the crew that just arrived at the hall enters the station and begins talking to Jake and Julie.

As I take a seat on one of the couches, the paramedics start telling stories about being "cold cocked" – that is, being hit unexpectedly by a patient. Julie turns to me and says, "We've all been assaulted on the job." Julie and Jake then tell a story of their own where Julie had to practise some "street medicine" when they came into contact with a patient who, according to Jake, was "kind of an ass ... [was] partying ... all night" with his son, who was "intoxicated ... got canned." Julie interrupts and says, "You missed me reading that guy the riot act [*laugh*]." She explains how they arrived at the scene and entered the house and both the son and the father were "being an ass ... I think I told the son three or four times, 'Stand back.'" She goes on to describe the following sequence of events:

> I tried to get the guy to come upstairs with me. And I go, "Seriously, come
> upstairs with me [*in a stern voice*]," and he goes, "You can't tell me what to

do. This is my house [*in a loud voice*]." And I just, I puff up like a fucking turkey and I can't remember what I said but it was something along the orders of, "[*yelling*] As soon as your father fell down the goddamn stairs, you lost control. Get your ass upstairs before I ... " And he was like, um, and he went up the stairs. And then he gets to the top of the stairs and he turns around and I'm at, it had like uh a stairway, a landing, and a little area where it changes angles, and a little flight of three or four stairs, and he gets to the top of those stairs and I'm still on the landing and he turned around and his mouth was open – he was going to say something – and I went, "[*yelling*] Don't you ever talk to me like that again [*Jake and the other paramedics laugh*]. If you ever talk to me like that again I'll flatten your ass and tear you a new asshole." And I just went up one side and down the other and all the firefighters down at the bottom of the stairs are all going ... and I went, "Now sit your ass down." He goes, "Yes ma'am."

Jake turns to me and explains how they often come into contact with people who are "belligerent, will try and kick us, punch us, stab us, shoot us. Uh, grope you. Make sexual comments ... and [*in a serious tone*] that's a no-no on my truck ... I've pulled over the truck, I got back there, I grabbed the guy, 'Touch my partner, say one more thing' [*laugh*]." Julie says that in order to protect yourself on the streets, you have to be "close enough to do your job, far enough to be safe." I ask about how this skill is learned, and Julie says that all it takes is the first time of being cold cocked to learn the need to protect yourself. Julie also says that sometimes you will see her abruptly pull her students away by the collar and explain to them that their safety was jeopardized. She goes on to explain that this method of teaching is necessary but sometimes scares students.

Part of what paramedics do is continuously orient to the non-standard nature of their environments. Julie's storytelling exemplifies this as she explains how she orients to her setting of a narrow staircase, a drunk patient, and concerns for her own safety as she proactively "defuses" the situation. This storytelling of being cold cocked and having to "lay down the law," because "we're in frickin' Kosovo here or Afghanistan downtown, you know uh, it's a war zone," is another part of what Jake and Julie described as "street medicine," which makes what paramedics do unique among health care professions. I was curious how this story got recorded in the ePCR so I asked Julie and she said, "Hostile environment."

Throughout my observations, storytelling was pervasive. Such storytelling occurred mostly at the station, in the ambulance, and in the garage or the halls of the hospital. Most research that examines talk as storytelling focuses on how paramedics use storytelling as a strategy for coping with their work. I viewed storytelling a bit differently, as an avenue to understand what paramedics actually do and how they understand their work. While I discuss one component of storytelling in this chapter, the storytelling that I heard throughout my research covered many facets of paramedic work and can broadly be thought of as teaching and learning. Viewing storytelling this way, we see how a central part of paramedics' work of learning occurs informally through telling stories and talking to colleagues on the front lines. One paramedic gave an example of teaching and learning work through storytelling: "We tell the stories that are funny or whatever, we ask 'What did you do?' 'What didn't you do?' 'How did the patient respond?' 'How did this happen? 'I'm not sure how to treat this. Have you had a similar situation like this?'"

"That Was a Gooder"

As the storytelling continues among Jake and Julie and the other crew, it seems as though they are competing for the "best" or "most shocking" stories about being cold cocked. This "jockeying"[1] is interrupted by the ringing of the tones. Julie and Jake quickly rise from their seats; Julie puts a lid on her container and places it in the fridge. Julie and Jake then quickly walk out to the garage with their coffees in hand, I follow them out to the ambulance, and Jake hops into the driver's seat and Julie into the passenger seat. We quickly exit the station. I hear something about chest pain and get a quick glance at the CAD screen that says, "Mom experiencing chest pain," but because we are driving hot with the sirens blaring and the lights glaring, I cannot hear what Julie and Jake are discussing.

No more than five minutes after leaving the hall, we arrive at what looks like an apartment complex. Julie grabs the red bag and Jake grabs the oxygen tank, blue bag, and Lifepak. I ask Jake why he is grabbing the blue bag, and he says that there is "no status on the patient" and he does not want to come back down to the ambulance if he needs the bag. Jake then makes his way to the exterior of the ambulance, places the supplies on the ground, and pulls out the stretcher. Once the stretcher is out of the ambulance and in the transport position, he places the supplies on the stretcher and follows Julie into a four-story apartment complex. As we are walking to the complex, a middle-aged man, the patient's son, I presume, meets us with the keys. We enter the building and then an elevator that barely fits the stretcher, let alone three adults (the son does not come in the elevator with us), though we shuffle our bodies and make it work. Once in the elevator, Julie presses the button for the third floor. This is followed by the doors closing, the elevator quickly rising, a soft jolt that slightly shakes my body as the elevator comes to a stop, and the doors opening. I follow Julie and Jake around a few corners and we arrive at a room with a door that is slightly ajar. Julie enters and identifies herself as EMS. Jake places the stretcher outside of the room and begins talking to the same man who was downstairs with the keys. As he is talking to the son, he pulls out the ePCR and begins asking the son about his mother's past medical history. He specifically asks him if she has had "issues with [her] heart." While Jake is talking to the son, the son quickly goes into the room and hands Jake a bag of the patient's medications.

I then direct my attention to Julie, who is in the patient's room asking her questions. Julie asks me to stay outside the room; presumably she is attaching the ECG leads while the patient is still in bed. It appears to me that Julie is doing her "standard" assessment when she suddenly leaves the room, approaches Jake, and shows him the ECG printout from the Lifepak. As she hands Jake the piece of paper, she says, "I need to talk to the doctor." Jake replies that it looks as if there is an "abnormality … there might be some changes here." Jake's demeanour suddenly changes; he later tells me that after he read the printout, he became "a little bit more aware" and was "listening more, a little bit more there" just in case Julie needed help.

Julie returns to the patient's room. I look through the door of the room and see Julie on her cell phone. Julie later explains that she not only did an ECG through the Lifepak but also faxed the ECG to the hospital through the modem embedded within the Lifepak and consulted with a doctor over the phone. While talking on the phone, she gives the patient what I would later find out was aspirin. She hangs up the phone and Jake enters the room. Julie asks the son for a shirt for the patient so she can "cover up" and assists the patient with putting it on. Jake then picks up the patient's left hand, looks at her arm and hand closely, then places it down and does the same thing with her right arm. He then takes a syringe from the red bag and starts an IV on the patient's right arm.

While Jake is setting the IV, the patient tells Julie about frustrations with her past medical experience in the hospital, saying, "If I could throw spit balls of fire [at the hospital], I would." The patient expresses her desire not to go to the hospital. In response, Julie begins to convince the patient that she must. She says, "My love, if you were my mom, I wouldn't want you to stay at home." While trying to convince the patient to go to hospital, Julie asks the patient to lift up her tongue so she can spray some "nitro" under it. After Julie administers the spray, she presses her radio and says, "Dispatch, we're code 15." After some time, the patient reluctantly agrees to go to the hospital, though she says, "I am so frustrated." Julie then asks Jake and me to leave; "I'm going to get mom decent." Jake replies, "I'm going to get the stretcher ready."

From the patient's room, Julie asks Jake to "mark the nitro" in the ePCR, indicating that she has given the patient another dose. Jake then re-enters the patient's room, and I follow. Talking in front of the patient, Julie empathetically explains to Jake that "we have a frustrated lady here." Jake then leaves the room and continues his prepping work by adjusting the height of the stretcher, setting the buckles to the side and then pulling the sheets apart to prepare for the patient to sit on it. I also notice that he shuffles the bags around and moves the oxygen to organize his supplies. Julie then sits the patient up and wraps the blood pressure cuff around her arm. As she does this, I notice that the patient looks pale. Suddenly the patient starts to heave and Julie, in a loud voice, calls for Jake to "get in here."

Julie asks Jake for a throw-up bag. Jake quickly comes in the room with one, which is a bit late as only some of the vomit makes it into the bag. Julie says to the patient after the heaving stops, "Darling, you passed out." When I hear this, I feel my heart speed up and begin to pound. Jake quickly leaves the room and seems to be moving much faster. I notice that he begins to move stuff around in the apartment, such as a couple of chairs, a coffee table, and desk/mirror unit. Julie turns to me and asks me to get the red bag. As I rush out of the room, I hear Julie ask the patient if she knows where she is. As I bring Julie the red bag, I notice that she is on her radio with the Dispatch Centre. I would later learn that she was asking for medical backup, whereby another para-medic crew will join the call and assist as needed. Soon after this, Julie turns to the patient and says in a calm and reassuring way, "I want you to stay awake for me." Julie then repeatedly says the patient's name. Jake rushes into the room and asks me in a loud and serious tone that made sure I would hear him, "Mike, can you move the bed over there?" Jake would later explain that a "big part of our job is modifying your environment to suit the call ... there's aspects of the job that you don't know, when you go into school, like they don't teach you that. You're rearranging people's houses, you're movers, you're shakers [*laugh*]." He went on to explain how his work of modifying space, often with the intent of creating space, connects to the need to speed things up:

> When she went limp here and went unresponsive on us it was like holy cow. And then she wasn't coming out of it, then you start hustling. That's when you saw me grab the IV, grab this, move the bed. And then you're like, we're starting to think how are we going to extricate her. We have to figure that out so it's like well, we'll pull the bed, slide this down [the stretcher], throw her on and out the door.

Jake expands on this mental work:

> Our minds do go like holy crap. We start running through the scenarios in our head so. Yeah, our heart rate gets going up here ... you get moving and that. You start thinking and then your brain starts processing from the level, you know, low intensity up ... I have to start thinking, the next five steps, like I said, how are we getting her out of here, how are we getting her transported. So we start banging those things through our head ... She [Julie] took care of the patient mostly, I got the equipment and every- thing like that, she called for [medical] back up, I got the IV up. Your level does increase. You noticed that we were moving quicker here. We had to move quicker ... You just got to move quicker because time may be of the essence 'cause you just don't know what the heck is going on.

Before the patient is loaded into the stretcher, Jake explains to the son what happened: "OK, she's had a fainting episode here but she's responding to us now." He tells the son what hospital we will be going to and the son soon leaves. Jake then turns to me and says:

> [I] try and not do any yelling in the room, that gets people's heart rates up. Next you know ... They're in the way, and it gets their anxiety level, right. Uh, we try and talk at a low key, like no yelling. It does happen sometimes, sometimes you have to, you know your adrenaline level gets going ... You put on a front for them even though you're thinking in the back of your mind we have no idea what's going on.

With Jake's assistance, Julie loads the patient onto the stretcher. While doing so, Jake asks me to hold the IV bag and run to the elevator to press the button. We soon make our way to the ambulance. Once in the ambulance, Julie takes a seat in the airway chair, Jake sits on the sliding seat, and I sit opposite Jake. Jake hands me an IV bag and asks me to hold it. We immediately leave for the hospital "hot" – lights flashing and sirens blaring – with both paramedics in the back while one of the paramedics who was called for medical backup drives. As we are leaving, Julie jokingly asks the driver if we can stop for coffee.

On the way to the hospital, Julie asks the patient to squeeze her hands. After this, she takes out her cell phone, calls triage, and says something along these lines: "We're bringing in a code 1 patient." She then briefly tells the nurse about the patient's condition and finishes the call by saying, "ETA seven minutes." As Julie and Jake are opening up supplies and discarding packages on the floor, Julie turns to me and says, "This is the fun part. To make a mess." The patient is still passing in and out of consciousness. As the patient lies there unconscious, Julie attempts to insert a small tube in her nose but is unsuccessful. After she pulls the tube away, Jake looks to me and quietly says that the patient "didn't tolerate" the intervention.

Code Room

Once we arrive at the hospital, Jake and Julie quickly remove the patient from the ambulance and, walking at a much faster pace than usual, roll her past the triage desk and into what I later learned was the code room or trauma bay. On the way past the triage desk, Julie says to one of the nurses, "It's a little bit of a hm." Once we arrive in the code room, and with the assistance of hospital staff, the patient is quickly transferred to a hospital bed. There are about five people waiting around the code room. Soon after, about four more people arrive. After the patient is transferred to a bed, Julie begins to speak in a loud voice to what now appears to be at least 10 hospital staff, most of whom are gathered around the patient. I notice that about three or four of the staff are standing back, and two of them have their arms folded across their chests. I assume these are the doctors, as they are all men dressed in business casual attire, which is different from how the nurses are dressed. As Julie is talking about the patient's condition, I also notice that there is a nurse sitting on a stool taking notes.

After about two minutes of speaking to the hospital staff in the code room, Julie leaves and Jake and I follow. Jake explains that in the trauma room, you speak "loud, calmly, uh, and uh, and you try and keep your wits there like if it was a very busy call; you're trying to intubate here, do this, and get the whole story right in your mind." Julie goes on:

> One thing I say to students is "Do you know the story, before we get out of here and go to the trauma bay, do you know what you're going to say?" 'Cause a lot of the time you just don't just have time to think, so when you get in there you resort back to a certain, like, flow. It's like an algorithm, "OK, 45-year-old gentleman here uh, struck by a car while crossing the road, speeds around 50 kilometres per hour. He was thrown approximately 30 yards. Unconscious on scene and en route to the hospital. He's got obvious deformity to his forehead here, lower left leg fracture," bang, bang, bang, give your vitals. So it's kind of like our PCR form; we go from the history of the event, patient presentation, what you got for vitals, what you did type thing. So that's how I try and tell students, like do it in order … It can be extremely intimidating for students … That's why you just have a system; who do you have, what happened, what you found, what you did, any changes. If they want to ask you more questions, that's why you stick around. It's fun …

"On Our Truck, Everyone Is 36.5"

As we leave the emergency department and head to the ambulance, which is parked in the garage, Julie leans over to me and quietly says, "That was a gooder. I'm glad that you've finally got to see something, as awful as that sounds." She was referring to how, in her and Jake's opinion and that of many of the other paramedics I rode with, I was plagued by what they referred to as the "ride-along curse," resulting in my not seeing any "good" calls up until this point. I, of course, disagreed with this interpretation of what a "good" call was, because, as I explained to them, everything I saw was new, interesting, and therefore "good." Nevertheless, this discussion of good as opposed to shit calls and the ride-along curse connects to insights from Becker (1993), who discussed how this "crock of shit" talk – talk that health professionals use to distinguish between "classes" or qualities of patients – reflects the "interests" of the workers using such language (p. 31). In this case, I understood this talk to reflect the desire of paramedics to treat "real" or "true" emergencies or "interesting" calls. I also began to think that this language points to how these paramedics interpret and give meaning to their social world in relation to the quality of calls/patients they come into contact with, and also points to the socially organized character of their work settings.

While in the garage, I ask Julie and Jake to talk to me about different facets of this call. I first ask them to talk about their use of the Lifepak and how it interfaced with their work. Julie pulls out one of the printouts from the Lifepak and explains to me how her work orients to information produced by the Lifepak. Showing me the printout, which to me looks like a bunch of squiggly lines, she says:

> There's changes actually in here, these two, these two strips ... This is a twelve-second picture of a heart in time in three-second segments. And in each three-second segment uh there's twelve of them right. And in each three-second segment is showing kind of like a view, a certain angle of an area of a heart. And uh, what it shows is, we look for specific changes, like basically uh, you know they teach you how to read this but I see a couple things here uh in the ones that are labelled V1 and V2 uh that you could potentially get excited about and if these changes didn't exist in her old ECGs we could say she's actually having a heart attack. But these changes are old [according to the doctor Julie spoke with over the phone] so this is obviously some kind of pathology, which is normal for her in the presentation. So sometimes, like I could have potentially gotten excited about these [*pointing to the printout*] ... The doctor was like, "Uh, no" or he'll go "Holy shit, get them in fast," right. But um, I like to use that as a tool ... actually using the doctors as a tool. Do I get excited about this or no?

The ECG printout evoked parts of Julie's work as it did Jake's; in printing out the document and taking time to read it, both Julie and Jake oriented to certain information in it. Jake, for example, "listened" a bit more closely to what was going on, and Julie phoned a doctor. Julie contrasts this talk with doing CPR on a patient. She explains that when she does CPR, her work also orients to the Lifepak technology, although a bit differently. Looking at the screen of the Lifepak, which is similar to the ECG printout, and intermittently referring back to a recent experience of doing CPR on a patient, she explains:

> So the top, when you look at the ECG strip. On the top you'll see is his heart rhythm. So you'll have his heart rate and whatever the rhythm is

... It will be deceiving because you'll see our CPR. It will look like a very odd heart beat. You can see our compressions. And then you'll see every time we stopped, just for a few seconds, just to see if we had anything, and then continued. Below that you'll see that line you were talking about, and that's his end tidal CO_2. That helps us measure, we want it between 35 and 45, and that helps us measure how well he's being oxygenated. So if he has, if he's getting, you know too much oxygen and doesn't have enough CO_2 or vice versa, he has too much CO_2 – we're not bagging him properly – it's really good for us as to how well we're bagging him. Do we need to go slower? Do we need to go faster to make sure he is being ventilated properly?

Both paramedics are orienting to the biomedical knowledge produced through the Lifepak, though each might take it up differently depending on the context; the information produced while doing CPR and in the case of the person passing in and out of consciousness is central, though the information is taken up differently within each setting. According to Julie, the information produced through the Lifepak during CPR is informative about the quality of intervention the paramedic is doing. In contrast, the information produced through the Lifepak during the call of the patient passing in and out of consciousness is also important in how the technological information contrasts with how the patient was actually "presenting." This resulted in the paramedics calling the medical information from the Lifepak into question. Furthermore, in "consulting" with the doctor, the paramedics confirmed that the technological information produced via the Lifepak was "unremarkable," which was relevant for the current medical emergency.

In both examples, we see that the information produced through the Lifepak is not always clear-cut and there is work involved in filtering the information produced by the medical technologies and the information garnered from seeing and touching the actual patient. In other words, paramedics might rely on certain information produced by the technology while discarding other information depending on what information is being outputted but also depending on the context; rather than Jake and Julie solely trusting the information produced from different technologies, this talk exemplifies how they are at work skilfully interpreting this knowledge. Perhaps when I heard Jake joking with another paramedic that "on our truck, everyone is 36.5 [degrees Celsius]," which refers to the patient's temperature, he was alluding to how paramedics look beyond the face value of the information produced by the medical devices they use, the information dispatched to them, and even the information garnered from patients. Furthermore, Julie explained that the level of training and experience of paramedics might also play a role in how information is interpreted and acted upon. Paramedics skilfully interpret or, as one paramedic described it, take with a "grain of salt" the information that they collect or that is passed on to them. In doing so, paramedics are always orienting to the "what ifs" of the non-standardizable context in which their work occurs.

Treating the Patient, Not the Protocol, Not the Machine

As Julie and Jake are explaining how medical technologies interface with their work, an older paramedic comes up to us and tells Julie and Jake that they should talk to me about patient care versus protocol care. This paramedic is referring to the protocols or procedural standards that paramedics work with, as outlined in the orange book. As Timmermans and Berg (2003) explain, and as will be discussed further in chapter 7, protocols like these form the heart of evidence-based medicine because they attempt to prescribe the behaviours of practitioners by outlining which steps in a medical encounter are to be taken, depending on what specific criteria are met. Julie and Jake at first seem rather defensive in light of this comment. Julie lets out a nervous laugh and Jake explains that some view "protocol" paramedics as "cookbook" paramedics, which I understand to be a derogatory label; I think that they thought this paramedic was insulting them by insinuating that they were protocol paramedics and, therefore, not able to think on their own.

Nevertheless, the talk that follows is telling about their work and provides me with the opportunity to learn about the complex use of protocols and medical technologies, especially in contrast to how the protocols are depicted in the protocol book (as relatively simple depictions of what to do depending on the chief complaint) and how paramedic work, as it interfaces with the protocol book, is written up in the ePCR.[2] Julie explains that "protocols are the official, by the book, way they want uh, want you to deal with a certain situation … So that's protocol care is what they, they give you a specific ah situation and they want you to solve it this way."[3] A field trainer who is responsible for training paramedics, and who is also a paramedic, explained that protocol use in practice is much more complicated because "what you'll find is that a patient doesn't just plant themselves on one protocol."

You know it's like you can read about epilepsy, but here's this patient that has epilepsy, but they're also diabetic and they could have a seizure because their blood glucose is low or they could be having it because their [*inaudible*] level's low, you know, never just one, right? So, the evidence-based protocol is great because ... you've got evidence that suggests that your treatment is the best possible, you know, and it's been studied against many different patients, but here you've got a complex person, right, they're not just one disease process, right, there could be co-morbidities that we're dealing with.

This complexity of the job, according to Julie and Jake, was reflected in the new provincial protocols, which they described as being more "flexible" than the older protocols because the new protocols "give us a lot more leeway to work more grey into the black and white." Julie gives an example of how protocols are used in practice by referencing the use of the pulmonary edema protocol:

Say if someone comes to you and they're presenting with pulmonary edema, which means they have fluid backed up into their lungs and they're not breathing properly, we're supposed to do nitroglycerin [*makes the sound of a spray*] under their tongue and then max that out and then go to ah, what's called CPAP, and then go to the patch and what not. We had a gentleman, if we had waited to go [*makes the sound and gesture of spraying nitro*] and used the protocol as it was in the black and white uh, he would have continued to deteriorate and we would have had to tube him and we would have had to breathe for him, and that's a very, very bad thing. So we actually bypassed giving him the initial treatment of the nitroglycerin and threw the CPAP on him, which is what he needed. So the protocol gives us the flexibility to go, "No, no, no, no, no, this is not good, and this is not timely, and this man is in a lot, and this dude was in a lot of trouble" ... we still used the protocol but we altered it. He still got the, the medications, he still got the protocol but instead of going ABC, we went BAC.

Jake explains that the "average call" is set up the way it is laid out in the protocols. But, according to Julie, the "preferable flow" is not always "feasible or realistic" based on how the patient is presenting. In fact, Jake explains that the "protocol algorithm is set up to have to escalate your treatments based on a worsening of the patient's condition." Depending on the acuity of the patient (e.g., difficulty breathing compared to "severe respiratory distress"), treatments might have to be escalated and "steps" in the protocol might need to be skipped because "I have to treat what I am seeing." We see in this talk that Jake and Julie flex or bend the protocols based on what they deem as necessary to meet the patient's needs. In the actual protocol (see figure 4.1), the word "consider" is used throughout ("consider CPAP at 5 cm," "If systolic BP less than 90 mmHg: Consider," "If no improvement: Consider," etc.). This language use is meant to reflect the flexible intent of the protocol and is in contrast to the previous protocols that were more "black and white."

In addition to flexing or bending the protocols based on how the patient is "presenting at the time, whether … little sick, medium sick, or really sick type of thing" (Julie), Julie says that paramedics also "adapt [their] treatments" by "combin[ing]" or "manipulating" the protocols. Julie depicts this by referring to the past call, where she originally treated the patient using the "cardiac" protocol "for a while," but when the patient became "syncopal" (she was passing in and out of consciousness), Julie stopped the cardiac protocol because the drugs that she was using based on that protocol could actually do harm. Jake jumps in to say, "You mix and match stuff when you have to" based on "sound paramedic judgment … We go through three or four algorithms on a patient with a belly pain that's nausea and vomiting. We treat him for various different things – you have to combine." Jake mentions how it "does say in the protocol book, when in doubt, you have to use your judgment … sound paramedic judgment supersedes a lot of this 'cause the protocols cannot answer every single question." Jake is alluding to how each protocol begins with a standard box that reads "Standard Approach and Ongoing Assessment," which is a very broad protocol that, according to a former paramedic I spoke with, refers to their designated "competency profile for paramedics."[4] A medical director I spoke with explained this box in the protocols as follows:

> The first box would be something called "Standard Approach and Ongoing Assessment," which means whenever a paramedic goes to one of these calls they have a standard approach and they have ongoing things, so that would include measuring an oxygen saturation, listening to the chest, getting their history, getting their medication list, that's all their standard approach and ongoing assessment, that's box one … So, that's why we included that line at the beginning of every protocol, standard approach and ongoing assessment, and that means as a paramedic you have a skill

4.1 Pulmonary edema protocol

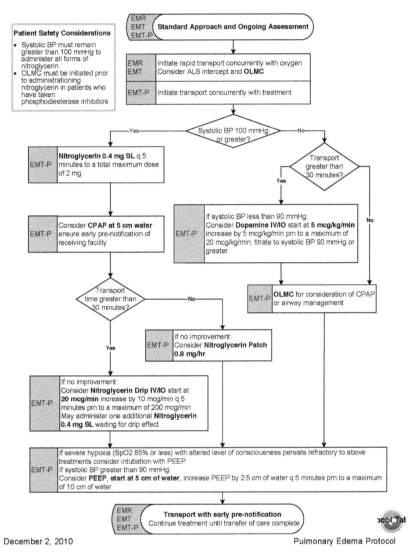

Pulmonary Edema Protocol

Source: © 2014 Alberta Health Services. See Acknowledgments for further attribution and disclaimer (2010a).

set that helps you determine what the patient's chief complaint or primary complaint is and what the highest acuity complaint is. So, nowhere in that manual do we say treat chest pain over shortness of breath or treat shortness of breath over nausea; we just, that's part of their base training that's in something called the core competencies document, that's a national document that says if you hold registration as a paramedic in this country, you will have this skill set for assessing patients.

Within this context of discussing the protocols, Jake explains that this ongoing assessment is part of the complexity and art of being a paramedic. According to Jake, it is the paramedic's job to do this interpretation work based on their "experience but also on patient care ... And that's when our training and our skills and our past history with other calls come into play." One of the medical directors I spoke with described this as "clinical acumen ... You can actually develop, pick and choose from the protocols which treatments are required for which patient based on their level of acuity ... That ability to pick and sort patients is developed with time and experience."

Treating the patient and not the protocol, or "machine," or "monitor," as other paramedics described it, is complicated by unclear "evidence" produced by medical technologies. Referring back to the last call, Julie says, "We can't explain what happened here. If it was simple, like her vital signs changed dramatically, then we can kind of treat that but when we don't see that, yeah we do get a little anxious ... " While paramedics rely on this technology to organize their medical interventions with patients, such technologies are not always clear-cut. Julie, thus, described the ECG printout as "disappointing" because it did not tell her much about the patient's condition – it did not show "a whole lot of abnormalities and that makes it really hard to diagnose." She goes on to explain how "you can figure out, if someone passed out because they were in this rhythm, when it's really blatant, but here she is in a normal rhythm with very minor changes to her ECG which are not new." We can see in this talk that Julie is looking for specific signs that can assist her in "diagnosing" what is wrong with the patient. This is what, in fact, made the call "interesting":

> So this was an interesting call because it had potential to be a stemi [heart attack]. If this was new [the ECG readings] we would have got excited about it but it wasn't new. But at the same time she had a change in her condition in front of us but we couldn't capture any changes [in the Lifepak] ...

Jake also explains how the technology often fails them because the design of the technology is not conducive to the complexity and non-standard nature of their work. Jake gives an example of a past call that I observed, where I noticed that he was having difficulties getting readings from the Lifepak, specifically the non-invasive blood pressure cuff. Jake explains:

> The patient, you saw her, she was moving around. The old fashioned way, we take our stethoscope and you pump up the cuff and you listen, well we like to cheat and speed up things [so] we'll use that [the Lifepak], and if the patient's moving around here or if it's a bumpy road, the cuff actually, it pumps up there and it detects the pulse … [but] if you're moving around it has a hard time picking it up so you get weird numbers. So that's why a lot of the time you have to tell people, "OK, just keep your arm nice and straight here." It's a technicality with the machine and sometimes they're not very reliable. Most of the time they are.

I heard and saw similar challenges with the ECG, which the paramedics refer to as "artefact." For example, while riding in the back of the ambulance to the hospital with a patient connected to the Lifepak, I noticed that the lines on the ECG machine monitor moved with the movement of the ambulance. When the ambulance was stopped, the lines were very smooth; when the ambulance went over a bump, even a small one, the curves on the monitor became less smooth. Figure 4.2 shows what I jotted down in my fieldnotes.

Jake and Julie orient to information produced by different technologies with skilful doubt, specifically being aware of "weird" information – information that starkly contrasts with other information they have collected (e.g., information from the actual patient). Julie explains to me that problems emerge for paramedics when they get "fixed on the numbers" or "treat the numbers instead of the patient or they treat the machine as we call it." Julie goes on, "So you have to be very confident in your ability to tell and look at the numbers that come up and say, 'I don't trust that' or 'Yes, I do trust that.'" Jake explains how he tries to teach his students to treat the patient and not the technology by having them "take away the blood pressure cuff. Do it the old fashioned way … don't get fixated on the monitor. Screw the monitor. The monitor is only telling us a few things here, treat your patient.' 'But it says this.' 'Fine, but how are they presenting?' 'Cause that's just a piece of electronic equipment … these things are built not for us but for the hospital."

4.2 ECG artefact

Ambulance stopped

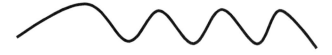

Ambulance going over bumps

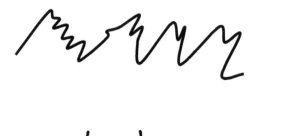

| Under the middle line was this line, which is how it looked when the ambulance was not moving. | This is how the line looked when the rig was bumpy. This is an example of "artefact." |

The "Social Stuff"

While the medical devices and protocols are standard, Jake says that, in addition to the reasons discussed above, their use is not standard because "it's very rare" that patients are "textbook." Patients are varied, Julie and Jake explain, and while medical technologies and protocols are there to help paramedics in their work, there is danger in solely trusting such technologies, especially considering that "patients with the same condition can present completely differently ... and your treatments can differ ... " (Jake). In fact, it is in this part of Jake's and Julie's job that they differentiate between protocol care and "then there's how you do the job" (Jake), much of which, according to Julie, consists of the "unwritten things that we don't get trained for but it's

80 per cent of our job." Julie is referring to the "social stuff" that they "don't get trained [for] ... they teach us the medical part." Jake expands on this by saying that his training taught him what to do on a call, but not how to "run" a call. Paramedics I observed exemplified this "social" aspect to their work when they described the different "hats" they wear as paramedics. Jake explained:

> You got to be a doctor, you got to be a police officer, social worker and uh, bad ass. A convincer. Sometimes you've got to coddle ... We do a lot of social work, and yes we treat medical problems and trauma problems but ... you're dealing with society here ...

Another paramedic explained what the "social stuff" includes:

> ... public safety officer roles, we have a little bit of psychology, a little bit of sociology, a little bit of home care, social work, all that stuff. And ah, 15 years ago, that wasn't in my scope, that wasn't in my mindset whatsoever and uh, I've been doing this for [over 15 years] and my brain has expanded and so has my scope. So ah, that's what keeps me here. You don't know what you're going to get. Every call is different. No two calls are the same.

While Jake and Julie discussed the need to use different parts of the protocol and mix and match other protocols, connected to this work is also the need to factor in the "social stuff," which inevitably interfaces with how they go about assessing their patients. Together, these interfacing processes exemplify the continuous assessment and constant vigilance work that is geared towards the "what ifs" of the realities of their work settings; Jake describes this work as "contingency planning all the time." In other words, in addition to orienting to what if "our treatments, if this doesn't work? What do I do? I have this many steps left on the protocol," paramedics orient to "the social stuff" and the variability involved with treating "non-standard" patients.

Self-Policing

Differentiating the old protocols from the new protocols, which Julie and Jake had just begun to use three weeks before my ride-alongs started, Jake explains, "The theory behind the protocols [is], especially these new ones, like Julie said, we're allowed to interpret them based on the situation ... They are more grey." Julie interrupts to say, "The

older ones, you know what, we did very well with the older protocols as well. They were much more cut and dried than the [new] ones
that the province has given us. The ones that the province has given us
are ... they are much more open to interpretation, and they are more
aggressive in our treatments of certain situations. I think they're a very
positive step." Jake adds that they are "good for us" because they allow
paramedics to work more to their full scope while recognizing how
medicine "is very grey." As such, paramedics are at work interpreting
the information that is created and output from these technologies and
interfacing this information with their own experience and training.

In addition to providing more "leeway" or "grey" areas in treating
patients, Julie says that the new protocols are also "more aggressive"
compared to the older city protocols. Alluding to their contradictory
consequences, Jake discusses these new protocols as a double-edged
sword. On the one hand, he explains that the new protocols are "good
for us" because they allow paramedics to work closer to their full scope
of practice. On the other hand, the new protocols increase paramedics' responsibility and potential for doing harm. A consequence of this
increased responsibility came to the fore during one of my observations
when Jake said to Julie in a serious but funny tone, "Don't make me
pull rank." This occurred when Julie was preparing to do an intervention on a patient that Jake felt was unnecessary. When I ask Jake to
discuss what I had observed, he describes this comment to Julie as an
instance of "self-policing." He explains:

> The protocols I think are going to save a lot more lives than the older ones.
> But that being said, we're going to have to self-police ourselves; watching
> myself, the two of us as a crew, and even watching other people and say-
> ing, "Whoa, whoa, should you even be doing that?" or "Hang on, hang on,
> why are you doing that?" We're going to have to be very, very diligent in
> that because we've gone from [being] handcuffed a little, and now we've,
> the leash has been lengthened on us so to speak ... This is all evidence-
> based ... There's a reason why we're doing this.

Expanding what paramedics in Calgary can do and what is expected
of them places more responsibility on them. While this is not necessarily
a bad thing, and most paramedics welcomed the additional responsibility, Jake voices some "chaf[ing]" (Rankin & Campbell, 2006, p. 74) with
this expanded scope when he expresses concerns that the new protocols
might create a situation where paramedics can do real harm to their

patients. In response to the new protocols, he discusses the additional work of self-policing and concern about treating the protocol rather than the patient, which connects to the discourse of providing the "right" care to the "right" patient at the "right" time. According to Jake, sometimes the "right" treatment for a patient can actually do harm.

At this point in our conversation, Julie is writing in her ePCR, and I notice that she has put three asterisks next to one of her comments. I ask her why she did this and she says that the asterisks are meant to draw the attention of the physician who is reading the document to something "really weird" that happened. Emphasizing the importance of the comments section for paramedics and other front-line workers, Julie explains:

> So if there's anything that I find extraordinary, either in a pertinent positive or a pertinent negative, or something that's just really weird, like outside the box, I'll always do that at the end of my PCR ... this happened or this didn't happen. You know like I put in here that I attempted to put in an NPA [the nose device] and she didn't tolerate it; that tells you a bit about her mental status ... she's more responsive to pain than I thought she'd be.

Fortying – "You Call, We Haul" – and Convincing Work

I sit in the airway seat, intermittently glancing at Julie filling out her ePCR. After about an hour, Julie suddenly leaves the ambulance only to reappear a few minutes later. She sits in the passenger seat and Jake soon follows. We leave the garage of the hospital and head back in the direction of the hall. On the way, Dispatch contacts Julie and Jake and asks them to "flex" to the south part of Calgary, as this part of the city needs "coverage." Flexing, I would learn over the course of my research, is a central part of "downtime"; it is a process whereby paramedics are dispatched to different areas of Calgary with the purpose of making sure "priority" areas of the city are "covered" based on a "flexible" deployment model that colour-codes each hall in the town, with red halls being more important than green halls. Because Jake and Julie are located at a green hall, "We're known as the flex truck for the city ... Dispatch will manoeuvre their resources around Calgary to make sure those [red and yellow] halls are covered ... Whereas if we were at one of these red halls when we come on for the day, we're basically there until we get a call. We're not being moved anywhere" (Julie).

While we drive to the south of Calgary, I have the chance to speak with Julie and Jake about something I have noticed throughout my ride-alongs with them and other paramedics: specifically, how the patient passing in and out of consciousness expressed her desire not to be transported to the hospital. The tone suddenly becomes more serious as Jake and Julie begin to discuss "fortying." Julie turns to me and says that fortying means to "cancel on a patient, which means we don't transport them. We go to the home, we assess them, uh maybe we treat them for something but then for whatever reason ... we don't take them to the hospital. We don't transport them at all. We leave them at home, often with instructions ... " Jake then interrupts and explains that their philosophy as a crew is that they do not cancel on the patient, patients "cancel on us."

> We, as a crew, that is our mandate. I've learnt from my other partners that, that's not our main goal is to cancel on people. They cancel on us. I assume that they're coming to the hospital until they say, "Well, I'm not going, I don't feel like it."

Jake then says, "We do forty a lot but, but I don't think our forties are unethical." Suggesting there is a right (ethical) and a wrong (unethical) way to forty, Julie and Jake discuss fortying in relation to their "mandate" as paramedics, which, according to Jake and other paramedics I spoke with, "is to transport people. You call, we're going to the hospital. I don't care if it's, my wig's fallen off, we're going to the hospital." Julie explains that if you approach every call with this mandate, "you should stay out of trouble because you're not jumping to conclusions – 'Oh, I'm going to forty on this bullshit.'" Even if the patient does not "feel like" going to the hospital, as explained above, paramedics work to convince their patients to do so. In fact Julie and Jake boast that they could count on one hand how many patients did not go to the hospital who, in their opinion, needed to.

I ask Julie and Jake to talk about this work of convincing patients that I had observed. This work involved not only convincing patients to be transported to hospital but also convincing patients to trust them. During one call, for example, a patient expressed to Julie, "I don't really trust medicine." After the patient said this, Julie seemed to orient to the patient's distrust of medicine, and told her in a very serious tone and looking directly into her eyes, "You have to be honest with me." This was followed by "I'm trying to help you ... You need to trust me, friend."[5]

Julie begins discussing convincing work with this brief story:

[I] went to a fellow who [was] having a heart attack and he refused to go, and my way to convince him was I said, "Well, I'll just stand here and wait for you to die then. And then when you die [*pause*] I have all the consent I need. And I will zap you back to life and then I'll take you to hospital." And he just kind of went, "Holy shit," and then he consented and I took him to hospital; he was having a heart attack and I had to be the biggest bitch to get him to go to the hospital with me.

Convincing work occurs within the context that paramedics cannot force someone to go to the hospital if "someone is completely cognizant, and uh, sound frame of mind ... That's kidnapping" (Julie). This was contrasted to "implied consent," where they can take people to hospital without consent who are either "unconscious" or "confused."[6] Also central to this work is the discursive context, which both paramedics and patients seemed to be aware of, that highlights how hospital emergency departments are experiencing major crises resulting in long and arduous wait times for patients and paramedics.

It is in this context of having to convince patients to go to the hospital that, according to Jake, you "see skills, my friend. Interpersonal skills. I think we're one of the best crews in the city ... I don't pat myself on the back a lot but Julie and I are very good at manipulating, convincing people, because a lot of crews will get to a certain point and then won't, you know what, we can turn it on when we need to; the charm or whatever we have to do." Jake explains that he tries to "make it personal" in an attempt to convince the patient; "You know what, I'm your friend here ... I'm telling you to go." Confronting the dominant discourse of hospital wait times, he goes on to explain how he will tell patients, "I don't tell you this because I want to sit in the frickin hospital hallway ... It's important enough for you to go."

Julie and Jake both describe how they use specific language to convince patients to go to the hospital. Julie exemplifies this by saying, "You know, the 'my dear' or 'darling,' 'my friend,' is always situation specific. Sometimes people are buddies, you know ah, especially the homeless guys, 'hey buddy,' you know, 'my friend' or something like that." Similarly, I had observed that while Jake was attending calls, he would often speak to patients using terms of endearment, especially when speaking with older patients: "my dear" (older woman) or "my friend" (male patients) in a soft and caring tone, which I heard continuously throughout my observations of this crew. This language use was specifically explained as creating an environment where the patient trusted Jake. Jake goes on to explain passionately:

> They say you're not supposed, I remember the studies that came out – "You shouldn't use terms of endearment" – you know what I've been doing this 10 years, fuck that ... I had [someone] chew me out one time on a call over that and I kind of had words with [the person]. I was like, "You know what, certain populations yes but with the older ones, you know what, I have never hurt anybody." It's worked for me for 10 years, 99.9 times out of 100, I will continue [to do] it. I don't care what some fucking study says about [it], I will do what I have to do to convince my patient to come, [even] if it's calling them "dear," "friend."

Julie discusses other convincing work strategies, such as using guilt-inducing language. Simply put, "I'll guilt trip them." (Jake: "Oh yeah"). In this context, Julie explains that she says things like, "If you were my dad, I wouldn't want you to stay at home." She also explains how patients would characteristically dictate exactly what she would say because "they always fall somewhere within a group that you can kind of touch at them a bit": "'If you were my grandma' or something like that, that works so well ... 'if you were my mom' or 'if you were my sister' or whatever I need to say to them." Both Julie and Jake describe convincing work as one aspect of "the art of this job" (Jake), whereas they describe the medical skills as the "monkey skills, they're basic."

This convincing work, according to Jake, is part of his "due diligence" as a paramedic and is organized by their current mandate of transporting patients. When patients are not transported, he explains, it is a "liability" issue. Immediately following this explanation by Jake, and alluding to changes that are "coming down the pipes" (Julie) and are connected to Alberta's new vision of health services that is geared towards putting the right service and patient "in the right place at the right time" (AHW, 2008b), Julie says, "I don't agree that every patient who calls us needs to go to the hospital uh ..." Referring to perhaps a changing of mandate, Jake says, "Until we're officially given that right ... I'm pretty hardball on that ... Until we have that legal protection, I don't cancel on patients. They cancel on me." Jake and Julie expand:

JAKE: And we're very, very careful on this car to watch how you say it. We work with tons of partners that say, "I don't think you need to go to the hospital."

JULIE: Oh, that is the worst thing to say.

JAKE: That right there, if there's a lawyer, the family's there, you are dead 'cause you've just, you've made that decision on behalf of the patient, and that's not in our mandate right now; we cannot say, "If you don't wish to go, here's some other options for you."

JULIE: I've actually said in front of my partner once, he told the patient that he didn't think that she needed to go to the hospital, and I told him I didn't agree. Right in front of the patient. I was like, "I'm not comfortable with that." And he said, "Well, we're not going to transport the patient." I said, "Well, you better damn well put in the document that I protested, because this woman needs to go. I can't believe you're saying she doesn't need to go."

JAKE: Like that right there, from a legal point, you're fucked. Absolutely fucked. The lawyers would rip you into shreds if something were to happen and that was recorded somehow or somebody heard that. "They said she didn't need to go."

While Julie and Jake are organized by their mandate to transport patients, Julie explains that she has a "mental checklist" that she goes through in every potential forty: "Can I leave them at home and be comfortable knowing that I've left them at home? ... If that mental checklist is an X then I'm going to convince them to go in." Jake adds, "We'll try and convince you ... If we think you do [need to go]." In other words, "If it's kind of a bogus call" (Jake) or what other paramedics described as a "shit" call, they might limit the amount of convincing work done.

Now, this convincing work did not occur with all of the paramedics I observed. One call with Dan and Hanna specifically comes to mind. We were called to a local bar because, according to the CAD, a woman fell and was bleeding from her head. Once the ambulance was parked, we entered the building, and Hanna approached the patient, who was lying on the ground, and asked her how many drinks she had had. The patient replied, "12 beer," in a slurred voice. After Hanna asked the patient some orienting questions, like what "day" and "year" is it and what "location" are we in, she gently placed her hands on the patient's head and looked briefly but intensely at the wound. Soon after, Hanna and Dan assisted the patient up and walked with her to the ambulance.

As the patient wobbled towards the ambulance, I overheard Hanna say to Dan that she "doesn't see a need for C-Spine."

Once in the ambulance, Hanna and Dan looked at the wound again and began to clean it with clear fluids and place gauze near the bottom of the patient's head to catch any liquid that would have otherwise dripped on her. In addition to tending to the wound, Hanna took the patient's blood pressure and measured her blood sugar. Hanna explained to the patient that she thought she needed a few stitches. Hanna then asked the patient if they could take her to the hospital. The patient said, "No." Hanna began to tap on the ePCR and, in a very calm way (to the point where I wrote down in my fieldnotes that she seemed "uninterested"), told the patient that she needed to go home if she did not "come with us." I remember being surprised by the lack of convincing work, work that I had been accustomed to seeing when riding with Julie and Jake. Hanna eventually asked the patient to sign the ePCR in a space that indicated that "you don't want to come to the hospital with us." The patient signed the ePCR and right after signing stated, "I'm drunk." Hanna asked a friend of the patient's who was standing outside of the ambulance to sign the ePCR as well.

While waiting for the patient to leave with the friend, who agreed to take her home, Hanna explained to her what she should look for with a head injury. She advised her to call 911 if she "throws up, feels numbness, [or] becomes dizzy." The patient soon left. We left the scene soon after but quickly pulled over to the side of the road so Hanna could finish writing the ePCR. I glanced at the comment section of the ePCR and saw that Hanna wrote the following: "Small Lace R Parietal of Head. No LOC, Pt is also x4. No Neuro deficit. Pt left with purse in hand." This "medical" or "disease" talk (see Frank, 1991) can be translated into the following: The patient has a small cut on the right side of her head. The patient had no loss of consciousness. The patient is alert to "the date, the time, the event, and who they are" (Hanna). The patient has no neurological deficits. Hanna also wrote in the comments section that the "patient repeatedly refuses transport to hospital." This last statement was contrary to my observations, as I had only heard the patient say "no" once. I wondered if what I observed on this call was an example of paramedics not convincing a patient to go to the hospital because they viewed the call as a "shit" call. I also wondered if the content written in the comments exemplified how paramedics sometimes use the comments section, as one paramedic had put it, to "cover your own ass."

On my current ride-along with Jake and Julie, we drive around the south part of Calgary for about 45 minutes, until the Dispatch Centre contacts us and says that we can go back to our station. Upon returning to the station, I exit the ambulance and thank Julie and Jake for letting me observe them for the morning. I say that I will see them in a week or so. They acknowledge what I say and voice and gesture a goodbye. I walk to my car and begin my drive home.

Chapter Five

Overview and Discussion
of Chapters 2–4

Overview

The longer I observed what paramedics were doing, the more "daz-zling" their work became (Giddens, 1997). In chapter 2, I discussed some of the work that goes into preparing and managing the ambu-lance for the day or night ahead, establishing and maintaining rapport while assessing and providing treatments to a patient, managing the scene, and writing up the work in institutionally appropriate and rec-ognizable ways. I also discussed the work of giving report to the hos-pital staff, specifically how paramedics orient to the work of the triage nurses when giving report, not only in providing the "right" informa-tion about the severity of the patient's conditions, but also in producing the "right" information in order to facilitate the allocation of emergency medical resources. I also brought to light some of the training and teach-ing work that paramedics do during their "downtime."

Chapters 3 and 4 provide additional descriptions of the work para-medics do on and off the streets. My goal was to expand on chapter 2 by providing layers of intricacies and messiness to what paramedics do. I described, for instance, the intricate work involved in medical devices and technologies. As an illustration, in chapter 3, in order to success-fully set up an IV in his patient, Dan orients to the possibilities of his patient pulling away and develops a work strategy for addressing this concern (e.g., "One, two, three, ouch, ouch, ouch"). We also see in these chapters that central to the "street medicine" paramedics administer is juggling between and filtering through the multiplicities of informa-tion they gather from many different sources, whether it be the patient, medical devices, and/or the Dispatch Centre. We see how paramedics read, understand, interpret, and call into question the medical technologies they work with and are aware that their settings (e.g., driving on a bumpy road or a patient being cold) can impact the quality of the information these technologies produce.

Much of the work of paramedics is geared towards and linked in text-mediated ways to the work of others in the EMS system, like EMS supervisors, dispatchers and call-takers, quality assurance auditors, and medical directors. For example, paramedics' link to others in the EMS system is facilitated by different interfacing technologies such as those at the Dispatch Centre (e.g., REPAC) and in the ED (REDIS and CTAS), and the ePCR and protocols. In addition, there are textual practices of accountability throughout the scenes described in the previous chapters. For instance, we see in chapter 2 that, in prepping the ambulance at the beginning of the shift, paramedics are supposed to sign a "Vehicle Check Sheet." Signing this sheet is a textual practice of accountability that is meant to ensure that the ambulance is in good working order. Julie explained that signing off on the sheet "is proof that the vehicle is ready for our um, string of calls."

A Reflection on the Diversity of Ride-Alongs

One of my goals in describing the three ride-along shifts featured in chapters 2, 3, and 4 was to shed light on the elaborate mental, physical, interpretive, and interactive work of paramedics. Nevertheless, the shifts and calls I have described represent only a snippet of my over 200 hours of ride-along observations and the many interviews I conducted with paramedics. During my observations, for instance, almost half of the calls I observed concerned seniors (42 per cent), and many of the patients I observed were of lower socioeconomic status. Furthermore, the diversity of calls I observed included "psych" calls, individuals experiencing "breathing problems," chest pains, nosebleeds, or drug overdoses, and calls where individuals were assaulted, in car accidents, suspected of having carbon monoxide poisoning, or "just fucking drunk."

In addition to this diversity, many of the calls, according to the paramedics I rode along with, were non-emergencies or what they sometimes called "shit" calls. For example, of the 59 calls I observed, only a few would have been classified by the paramedics I spoke with as "true emergencies" needing immediate medical intervention. In addition to the "gooder" call described in chapter 4, one of these calls was a "code 99," where the patient went into cardiac arrest and was not revived after attempts to "save" him, which included CPR and pharmacological interventions. Another instance was a "trauma" call, where the patient was severely beaten and needed immediate attention by paramedics and emergency department staff (see Corman, 2016).

Many of the paramedics I met would describe these few and far between calls as "gooder" calls. In fact, throughout my ride-alongs, many paramedics apologetically spoke of the "ride-along curse," a phenomenon where a shift was plagued by "shit" calls or "a lot of stupid flexes" because someone was riding along with the crew. Paramedics used this phrase as an explanatory tool for the lack of "good" calls that I was exposed to during my ride-alongs. Nevertheless, the demographic characteristics of patients and the types of calls I observed appear to represent the diversity of patients who visit emergency departments in Canada, at least based on the limited data available (Canadian Institute for Health Information [CIHI], 2005).[1] With that said, the number of emergent responses where paramedics drove with their lights and sirens on seemed to outweigh the actual number of emergent patients. In other words, calls seemed to be classified as more emergent from the Dispatch Centre than they were determined to be by the paramedics.

In addition to the types of calls and patients I saw, I was also able to observe different crews in different quadrants of Calgary, at different times throughout the year. This added to the complexity of my observations. Some crews, like Jake and Julie, had been partners for some time and had good rapport with each other. Other crews, however, might have only just met one another for the first time at the beginning of their shift or worked together only intermittently. Furthermore, Tammy, a paramedic for around 10 years, explained how EMT-Ps often have to "bounce" a lot, referring to being moved to different stations in Calgary so that each ambulance has an EMT-P on it, which is a requirement for the service to be designated an ALS service. Paramedics might have unfamiliar partners if someone was away or at another station and an "on-call" or "casual" paramedic was needed.

One of the on-call paramedics I observed and interviewed explained that such paramedics are used on a "short-term" basis to fill vacancies as needed because "guys like me, they pay me standard and I just get moved everywhere around the city." I asked this paramedic, "Do you get phoned the day you are working?" and he replied, "At times. Sometimes it's a month and a half in advance. Sometimes it's like, 'I needed you an hour ago.'" Julie, who was working with this paramedic as he was explaining to me how things work, said, "On-calls, they get screwed." The following conversation occurred:

M: Why is that?

JULIE: Well, they can work a lot of hours and not make overtime. And uh, they, the reason why they created the on-call list is because I'm expensive to pay double time. He's cheap to pay, regular pay.

M: So on-calls don't get overtime?

JULIE: They get overtime for the shift, like for the day, like everyone does. What happens is that they can work them five days in a row and not pay them overtime.

M: Do you guys get benefits?

ON-CALL: No. No benefits.

M: No health care or anything?

ON-CALL: No … No we get nothing.

M: And how new is the on-call list?

JULIE: The on-call thing has been going on forever. The on-call list dropped, it became really, really small a few years ago. But since the [provincial] government's taken over … the on-call list is huge. They have to fight each other for shifts.

ON-CALL: The summer's not the problem. Between this and my other job [as an EMT elsewhere] … I'm booked every day for a month and a half.

The use of on-call staff is a strategy aligned with neoliberal tenets "aimed at efficiency or cost-cutting" (Campbell, 2008, p. 278). One hidden danger of using on-call staff is that it could create a situation where the partner work described in these chapters was not developed, or distrust, rather than trust, was at the centre of the work relationship. As a case in point, I remember one ride-along in particular when Julie was partnered with an on-call EMT whom she had not worked with yet. As the shift went on, I could tell that Julie was frustrated with her new partner, as indicated by intermittent eye-rolling, and, having ridden along with her many times before, I could also tell that she was frustrated by her tone of voice. I asked her to talk about being partnered with a paramedic with whom she had not previously worked, and she explained, "I don't like it," because she does not "know how good they are or are not." She went on to explain that she "watch[es]" the paramedic until she decides "whether or not I like them." I asked her what she looks for in making this determination, and she explained, "I want someone who's competent and someone I can at least, that I don't feel like I need to treat them like a student." In terms of being "competent," Julie is concerned about working with paramedics "that you've never worked with before and you don't know what their skills are. Right, especially with the on-calls ... some on-calls, you see them a lot and you get to know them and other on-calls you've never seen them before." Julie also spoke about the reputation that different on-call paramedics are labelled with: "Some on-calls, because they work so often, they get reputations. Good reputations and bad. There's some people where you hear a name and you go, 'Oh, I'm so sorry.' Or other people, you hear a name, and you're like, 'Oh, that's good. Cool, you'll have an easy night.'" Based on what I heard and learned from paramedics, it appears that their work setting is increasingly being organized by interests geared towards flexibility rather than continuity (Campbell, 2008), with significant consequences both for workers and potentially for patients; as we saw in chapter 2, the partner work of paramedics is integral to patient care.

The location of where the crew was stationed in Calgary also structured, in part, the types of patients and calls they would be more likely to see, which may invoke additional complexities in paramedics' work practices. For example, the northeast and southeast parts of Calgary, which were referred to by more than one paramedic as "the ghetto" or "the hood," are more culturally diverse than the northwest and southwest parts. These eastern quadrants are made up of more visible minorities of lower socioeconomic status, which added complexity to paramedics' work, especially for paramedics who found it challenging to communicate with individuals whose first language was not English or who had culturally different backgrounds from their own.

Complexity was also evident in the northwest and southwest parts of Calgary, where seniors could make up many of paramedics' patients. Many paramedics I observed spoke of seniors with contradictory ageist undertones, as expressed by one paramedic who used the acronym "BTS. Born too soon," while also using a language of endearment when she said, "I love dealing with the gerries." Julie explained that seniors are "the majority of our calls" and they are challenging and "difficult medical cases [*laugh*], you know they're on fifty different types of medicines, fifty different types of medical problems, and that, trying to figure out what happened." When working with seniors, paramedics might orient to and may be aware of certain medical conditions and "Goals of Care Designations." The "Goals of Care" designation document legally organizes the type of medical intervention paramedics and other health care practitioners can do to a patient. The only time I saw paramedics ask for this document was when their patient was a senior. Julie, for example, explained that if the paper is not present on the scene, "I have to attempt full life-saving measures because it's implied consent ..." In contrast, if the patient has the document on their person, depending on the patient's designation, the types of interventions that paramedics can and cannot do are limited. For some designations (e.g., C1 and C2), the paramedics might have to watch the patient "die" as they transport them to hospital, "and there's nothing you can do," except "symptom control" to manage pain. Working with seniors may also include using different speaking styles and being more aware of specific social issues that pertain to them (e.g., elder abuse).

The diversity of calls in the four quadrants of Calgary can be further contrasted with crews working in downtown Calgary. These "city centre crews" seemed to come into contact with individuals who often use EMS, known colloquially as the "frequent fliers." In or near downtown is where homeless shelters and other social service facilities geared towards persons in need are located. As a result, city centre paramedics interfaced with this social context and these institutional services of support and were therefore more likely to treat what some paramedics referred to as "high-risk clientele" or "urban outdoors men." In fact, Calgary has specialized crews who have a different set of standard operating procedures, which allow them to give treatments, make referrals, and do "high risk cancellations" that are otherwise not allowed in Calgary. Of course, it was common for crews from one section of Calgary to be "pulled" into another part when sections of the city were "fall[ing] apart" and needed coverage. Therefore, while I provide a reflection on the breadth of calls that I observed, adding to the complexities and uncertainty of paramedics' work is the need to be prepared to work in any section of Calgary at any given time.

Orienting to the "What Ifs"

As my observations and interviews unfolded, I began to see how paramedics often use specialized knowledge, garnered from on-the-ground experiences, that informs their work in complex ways. For example, I soon realized that paramedics sometimes orient to and make assumptions about their patients, which, combined with the location of the call, notes from the Dispatch Centre, categorization of the call, and so on, can organize their work processes. I began to think of this work as prejudging work, often based on social categories like age, class, race, ethnicity, and gender. With that said, if my observations and interviews taught me anything about what paramedics do, it is that despite being able to respond to what may appear as "similar" calls and "similar" patients, paramedics orient to the contextually varied and non-standard aspects of their work. For example, paramedics spoke of "good" and "shit" or "asshole" calls throughout my observations and interviews.[2] While they are able to differentiate calls based on what may or may not be an exciting, difficult, and challenging call, or a patient with, as one paramedic put it, "a stuck fart ... That's my generic, 'You've called EMS for what?'" paramedics' work is geared towards the non-standard potentiality of their patients and work settings.

The complexity of paramedics' work is exemplified by how their work processes gear towards the "what ifs": the potentiality of their patients, the scenes, and the different information and communication technologies they use. This orientation was exemplified when Jake and Julie (chapter 4) spoke about bending or shifting between protocols, or by the constant vigilance of paramedics as they continuously orient to the non-standard potentiality of their work (e.g., being "cold-cocked") and gear towards the immediate, yet unplanned and multidimensional, nature of EMS calls and their patients. I began to think of this work as Jake summarized it: "It's predictably unpredictable."

The work of paramedics, as described in chapters 2–4, is complex and messy; it changes and adapts to emergent and unpredictable patients and environments. While paramedics' work processes are messy, these processes are also skilfully structured by the contours of paramedics' work settings, experiences, and training and how they continuously react to the complexity of their patients and the knowledge produced via information and communication technologies. I began to see stretcher work, for example, as a microcosm for other complex, yet structured, work processes, such as prepping the ambulance, treating patients, partner work, working with medical devices (e.g., Lifepak), or interfacing with medical and institutional technologies. Until I observed the artful work of loading a patient onto a stretcher, I had assumed that lifting, transporting, and loading patients were all simple tasks. After observing this work, I gained a more multifarious understanding of what paramedics do to successfully lift a patient and transport and load them safely. Also, institutional factors, such as how stretcher design favours a taller and perhaps a stereotypical male physique in a carrier, impacted stretcher work. What became obvious after observing the work of paramedics for an extended period of time was that their work processes were not linear but rather occurred within ongoing social historical processes. Smith (2005) uses the term *ongoing social historical processes* in recognizing the social as happening. She writes, "Each moment of action is conditioned by what is historically given and reshapes the already given in moving into the future" (p. 70).

Taken-for-Granted Work: What Counts and What Is Being Counted

Before I began this research, I took much of the work described in the chapters for granted. I would later learn that much of this work is also taken for granted and/or assumed by others in the health care system, perhaps necessarily at times, and particularly by the people who rely on the information produced by certain technologies central to how front-line EMS work is made visible in order to produce further information that is commensurable and "objective." One paramedic best described this line of fault when he explained to me that, since Alberta Health Services took control over Calgary EMS, "We're being run by people who have no idea what we do ... we have less voice than we've ever had before." This is important because this complexity is filtered out of the purview of what "officially" counts on the front lines of EMS. While some of this complex work interfaces with and gets recorded by institutionally mandated policies and practices, we will see in part 2 of this book how much of what paramedics do is unrecorded – many of the work processes of paramedics described in the previous chapters get written out of the different technological devices used to represent official understandings of their work. So what? What gets counted, vis-à-vis different textual technologies, institutionally measures what counts for administrators, managers, and policy makers, which has implications for the work of patients, front-line health care workers, and how the health care system is targeted by reform and restructuring practices.

I began to think of this complex work, and how it was rendered (in)visible from afar, as representing another microcosm of how knowledge is being put together on the front lines of EMS; much of the work paramedics do is central to their own everyday lives and those of their patients, yet it goes unrecorded and unrecognized (Diamond, 1992). How Jake and Julie orient to the medical devices and call them into question, and how they use the protocols, reflects the complexity of this work, yet this complexity is wrapped up, assumed, and subsumed into a very broad category that exists in every protocol as "Standard Approach and Ongoing Assessment." I began to see that much of the work that paramedics do during a call is encapsulated in this very broad category; it takes up "the bulk of the day and constitute[s] the most complex part of the work" (Diamond, 1992, p. 131), yet there is no corresponding box or category to be filled out in the ePCR, except, perhaps, parts of the comments section. The solution is not more or better boxes per se but rather a more in-depth understanding of actual work processes and the socially organized setting in which that work occurs in order to develop a different mode of knowledge that adds to and sometimes challenges "knowing in text-mediated ways," which is integral to relations of ruling (Campbell & Gregor, 2002, p. 36).

Furthermore, what gets counted institutionally is not necessarily the same as what counts for the paramedics. For example, the work that gets written into the quantified and reportable categories of the ePCR is characterized by a process where the work of prejudging, convincing, and modifying space is subsumed into specific institutionally recognized information (as will be seen in chapter 7). The section that seems to really count for paramedics – the comments section – is discursively organized by biomedical, accounting, and legal logics, and does not get counted in the same way that other sections of the ePCR do, though it is potentially used by physicians, lawyers, and as we see in the next chapters, some other players in EMS.

We see in chapters 2–4 that what gets known institutionally is socially and discursively organized by different technologies that either enter into the work of paramedics (e.g., protocols) or quantify certain aspects of their actualities (e.g., ePCR). What is important here is that such technologies, by the very nature of how they are designed and the purposes for which they are used, necessarily capture and represent only snippets of what actually happens. Building upon chapters 2–4, the chapters that follow continue to problematize this demarcation between what is known institutionally and "systematic practices of 'not knowing'" (DeVault, 2008, p. 290). In other words, the knowledge produced through the different technologies that interface with the work paramedics actually do and the accounting of their work institutionally is only the tip of the iceberg, so to speak, of what is actually happening on the front line.

Other Players in Emergency Medical Services

Part 2 provides a more in-depth analysis of how the work of paramedics is put together, made visible in the age of technological governance, sometimes with hidden consequences. My goal is to begin to unpack some of the institutional relations embedded within the descriptions of the everyday work of paramedics that have been the focus of chapters 2 through 4. In chapter 6, I focus on the work that occurs in the Dispatch Centre. I view this institutional site of coordination and control as a processing interchange that interfaces with the front-line work of paramedics, specifically geared towards the efficient use of pre-hospital resources. Whereas chapter 6 explores technologies that target the efficient allocation of emergency medical space and "labour resources" (Rankin & Campbell, 2006, p. 85), chapter 7 explores technologies of knowledge and governance that are targeting clinical practice and knowledge production practices central to accountability and quality improvement projects.

These latter chapters blend together in explicating the textual representations geared towards reforming health care, and more specifically health care work, on the front lines of emergency medical services. In other words, the knowledge passed on and processed to other sites via the Dispatch Centre and the ePCR, and the information processed by the ED, all become "key organizational element[s] in taking action" and are the institutional representation of what counts, which ultimately "reflects the concerns of the institution" (Pence, 2001, p. 203). The analysis I undertake offers a different sort of empirical evidence from that offered by a textual representation of health care: evidence located in the actualities of people's everyday lives. This evidence has the potential to inform and challenge, and to make reform practices more generous and reflective of the everyday work of front-line workers, ultimately leading to more meaningful reform for front-line workers, patients, managers, and policy makers.

PART TWO

PART ONE

Chapter Six

The "Brains" of EMS

If you were to ask the paramedics what should we be studying right now, a lot of them would probably say the REPAC system, because you know a lot would say it probably sucks … I talk to a lot of paramedics and I know that there's a lot of issues with REPAC … Obviously the reason we do it is for efficiency, for effectiveness … I think that as a paramedic when I was out on the street, you know, one of the biggest things is that you get told what to do a lot … That's why a lot of paramedics are very picky about their ambulances and their world, because that's what they control, but there are a lot of external influences that tell them what to do, so it's a real challenge … (Research Officer)

Introduction

Before a call is activated for paramedics, there are people at work. Central to how paramedic work is organized is the work of people and the technologies with which they interface at the Dispatch Centre – what one paramedic called the "brains" of EMS. The Dispatch Centre in Calgary is located on the second floor of an emergency services building near the centre of the city. The first time I walked in, I remember feeling overwhelmed, not by the number of people present, which might have been around 30, most of whom were tucked in behind their workstations, but by the vast amount of technology. Each workstation seemed to have at least four computer screens and radio noises, and bell-like tones were going off around me and the sound of typing was incessant. One call-taker I spoke with explained that the tones or beeps could mean "there is a new dispatch going on, or a unit is clearing, or there's an alarm, like a unit alarm." I noticed that some stations had lights located near the top of their terminals that were blinking. I would later find out that a blinking light meant that someone had phoned 911 and was waiting "in the 911 queue" (call-taker) for a call-taker to become available.

I spent about three weeks intermittently listening in on and observing the work of call-takers (otherwise known as Emergency Command Officers) and dispatchers. I interviewed call-takers and dispatchers about their work as I was observing them in an attempt to gain a better understanding of what their work processes actually involved and how their work interfaced with others in the emergency system. I was also interested in exploring how their work was put together – socially organized by different institutional technologies – and made institutionally visible. To help me connect the dots and gain a better understanding of this socially organized site of work processes, I spoke with call-takers and dispatchers about the institutional technologies they used, and I spoke with the managers at the Centre with a focus on how their work interfaced with call-takers, dispatchers, and paramedics on the streets.

The manager whom I first contacted for an interview about dispatch operations gave me a tour of the Centre. She explained that the Centre is separated into two sections, one side dedicated to police services and the other side dedicated to Fire and EMS, though both sides are located in the same general area. While I was walking around the Centre, I noticed that there were desks located in between the two sections, roughly in the centre of the room. I later found out that these desks are for the managers of the call-takers and dispatchers. For EMS/Fire, there are two managers on duty during the day shift and two on duty during the night shift, with one supervising the call-takers and one supervising the dispatchers. These desks have additional computers and phones on them. Directly across from the desks are very large computer screens attached to the wall. The person giving me the tour told me that the screens display the "grade of service … much to the chagrin of the staff," which includes information like the numbers of calls, calls waiting, and how long it takes to pick up the calls. As I learned more about the Centre, I began to understand these statistics as key performance measures. One call-taker explained them as follows:

OK, those big screens, what they are showing on there right now is the status of each one of these terminals in here, the call-taking terminals and the dispatch terminals; whether they're on, how long they've been on, ready, ready to accept a call, etc. So, any time you log out it doesn't go unnoticed.

As I continued the tour, I glanced at the computers on the Fire/EMS side of the Centre; some of the screens looked foreign to me, while with others I could discern some similarities with the CAD screens located in the ambulances, such as maps of Calgary with different colour-coded truck-shaped icons that I was told represent the status of the crews. Black means that the crew is at their station, green means that the crew is ready for a call, orange means that the crew is on their way to a call, purple means that the crew is transporting a patient, red means that the crew has arrived at the scene, and blue means that the crew is at the hospital. The status of the vehicles, I would later learn, is used to assist dispatchers in keeping track of and dispatching the ambulance resources in Calgary. During the tour, my informant pointed in the direction of the break room and told me that it "was the only place in the Centre" where the phones were not monitored.

Most sociological research that investigates the work of those in Dispatch Centres uses ethnomethodology's conversational analysis (CA) to explore the "joint interactional work" (Cromdal, Persson-Thunqvist, & Osvaldsson, 2012, p. 200) or "talk-in-interaction" between call-takers and callers and how this interactional work is coordinated vis-à-vis talk for the purposes of dispatching or not dispatching emergency services (e.g., police and ambulance services) (Whalen & Zimmerman, 1990, p. 467). Using audio recordings to investigate "natural" sequences of talk, researchers have analysed the talk between call-taker and caller with the goal of gaining knowledge of "some orderly features of initial emergency reports," in order to understand how the different positions and orientations of caller and call-taker are coordinated to achieve some successful or unsuccessful assemblage of an emergency account (Cromdal, Osvaldsson, & Persson-Thunqvist, 2008, p. 928; Cromdal et al., 2012).

Understanding how talk is coordinated between callers and call-takers at Dispatch Centres and describing how technologies shape the work of callers is important because there is much at stake during this interactional event, such as the appropriate coordination of emergency services. However, the studies reviewed above differ significantly from this study. As Smith (2005) explains, "Ethnomethodology's conversational analysis [conversational analysis] can be understood as investigating how people's ordinary talk is coordinated" (p. 60). In doing so, CA "cuts out pieces" of social relational sequences for scrutiny, without a focus on the social organization that coordinates such interactional events. By focusing solely on isolated units of talk for analysis, "ethnomethodology and, more specifically conversational analysis, differentiates talk from what becomes its context, relegating the latter to a region that its methods do not embrace" (p. 67).

The consequences of this cutting-out process are reflected in what the CA studies fail to examine, primarily: 1) the institutional environment in which the work of people in the Dispatch Centre takes place; 2) how institutional technologies deployed at the Centre organize and coordinate the work of those in the Centre and collect and report knowledge of that work; and 3) the *interfacing work* of call-takers and dispatchers. Therefore, my goal in this chapter is to bring to the fore what is left in abeyance in these CA studies. More specifically, I explore the work of people at the Dispatch Centre and the highly organized and coordinated environment in which they work. In doing so, I explore "what people are doing or what they can tell us about what they and others do and ... how the forms of coordinating their activities 'produce' institutional processes, as they actually work" (Smith, 2005, p. 60).

I begin with an overview of some of the "official" work of people in the Centre. I specifically focus on the technologies of governance that are deployed to organize and coordinate the work of Dispatch Centre employees, and also the paramedic crews on the streets. I then move on to a more in-depth examination of the actual work that goes on in the Centre. Again, I focus on how this work interfaces with that of paramedics. I end the chapter with a brief discussion and conclusion on how these technologies link to governance practices in the city and province.

EMD and ProQA – "911, for What City?"

Highly coordinated and organized work processes begin when someone dials 911, as "the number 911 is the first in a series of texts that will coordinate, guide, and instruct a number of practitioners ... " (Pence, 2001, p. 201). When an individual dials 911 in Calgary, they are connected to a call-taker[1] located in the Centre. The call-taker[2] typically answers the phone by saying, "911, for what city? Do you need police, fire, or ambulance?" If the caller says that she is in need of police services, the call-taker transfers the call to a call-taker specific for police services. If the caller specifies that she is in need of fire or an ambulance, the call-taker begins the work of evaluating the call.

Call-taker: [*Phone rings*] 911, for what city? [*Pause*] And do you need police, fire, or ambulance? [*Pause*][3] For what address, please? [*Pause*] OK, I'll need

that address one more time, please. [*Pause. Sounds of typing from call-taker*]
Yeah [*pause*], OK, and what's the phone number you're calling me from,
please? [*Pause*] Yes. OK, and tell me what's going on there today. [*Pause*]
He hurt his eye? [*Pause*] Uh, huh. [*Pause. Clicking of the computer's mouse
from call-taker*] OK, I've got the paramedics on the way. I need to ask you
some more questions, OK? [*Pause. Sounds of typing and clicking of the computer's mouse from call-taker*] Are you with the patient right now? [*Pause*]
OK, how old is he? [*Pause. Sounds of typing from call-taker*] Is he awake?
[*Pause*] OK. Is he breathing? [*Pause*] OK. Is he completely alert? [*Pause.
Clicking of the computer's mouse from call-taker*] OK, so what exactly happened to his eye? [*Pause*] OK, so [*pause*] No, I understand that, but what
exactly is it that happened? You said he's bleeding. Do you know why, like
did he get something in his eye? [*Pause*] OK, is his eyeball cut open or is
fluid leaking? OK. OK, you need to listen to my question, ma'am. [*The call-
taker is now enunciating her words very slowly compared to her previous talk*] Is
his eyeball cut open or is fluid leaking out of it? [*Pause*] OK, I understand
you said it's cut badly, is [*pause. Sounds of typing from call-taker*]. [*The call-
taker resumes the original speed of her talk*] So, it's the skin under his eye, not
his eyeball? [*Pause*] OK, paramedics are well on the way, OK? Just a few
more instructions here ... Thank you, bye-bye.

The work of taking calls involves asking the caller a series of questions and entering certain information into the computer. The questions asked are based on what is called a "cardset" or dispatch cards.
The cards used at this Centre (and many Centres in North America)
are developed by the National Academies of Emergency Dispatch and
are called Emergency Medical Dispatch Protocols (EMD protocols). The
first set of "entry level" (call-taker) questions is intended to get contact
information so that the paramedics know where to go. The second set
of questions – "tell me what's going on there today" – is meant to identify the "chief complaint" that corresponds to one of the 33 cards that
make up the cardset.

Once a chief complaint is identified, the call-taker flips to the card that
corresponds to the chief complaint, which "usually correlate[s] with the
caller's primary complaint ... So, for instance, if we have a caller calling
in about chest pain ... we know right away we can go to number 10 card
that correlates with chest pain" (call-taker). Each card has additional
questions relevant to the chief complaint that are supposed to be asked
"verbatim" by the call-taker. Based on the caller's responses to the
questions, information is entered into the call-taker's computer, which

does two things: 1) "determines the levels of response" for paramedics (e.g., lights or sirens or cold response) (call-taker), and 2) with the click of some icons on the screen by the call-taker, information "populates" into the computer of the Alpha 1 dispatcher, who dispatches the closest unit to the scene. Some of this information also appears on the CAD screen in the ambulance.

The cards and computer in front of the call-taker mediate the talk and information produced and passed along to the dispatchers and eventually the ambulance unit(s) that will respond to the call (Pence, 2001, p. 201). The call type – the response determinant (e.g., Alpha, Bravo, Charlie, Delta, and Echo) – and the categorization of the patient into cards are supposed to reflect "risk" to the patient. For example, each card has certain "drivers" that dictate the categorization of the call and the call type. As one call-taker explained, "Bravo they'll go hot, Charlie they'll go hot, Delta they'll go a little bit hotter ... And then Echo, they're really on their way." Certain call types activate additional resources, such as whether the fire department will be dispatched and whether EMS supervisors are notified about the call. Similar to Case Mix Groups discussed by Rankin and Campbell (2006), the classification system of EMD Protocol is geared towards classifying patients with similar conditions and theoretically parallel resource requirements.

While paramedics orient to this information, specifically if they drive hot or cold, how they orient to the information is not so straightforward (see chapter 2). Information from the Dispatch Centre, for instance, is sometimes called into question by paramedics on the streets. One paramedic explained, "A lot of times, it could be a 26 Alpha [sick person], I'll still take all my stuff because there actually have been 26 Alphas that turned out to be cardiac arrests [an Echo call] ..." Conversely, paramedics orient to the possibility of a call being categorized as a cardiac arrest (Echo) and ending up being a person who is sleeping. As such, paramedics seem to orient to more than the information from the Centre, such as past experiences, time, day, location of the call, and notes about the call from Dispatch. The call-taker, on the other hand, is primarily orienting to the information garnered from the caller. As we will see later, this is what makes a "good" call-taker, at least institutionally.

In addition to classifying patients, the protocols are geared towards two endeavours: 1) minimizing the amount of time it takes to classify and dispatch services, and 2) ensuring that the information produced by the call-taker from the caller is as "evidence-based" as possible. The former endeavour has at its core the management of time because *time is of the essence* in emergency contexts,[4] a theme reflected in one call-taker's explanation that "we actually have 30 seconds to get an address verified, a phone number verified, and a call type put in to get an ambulance or a fire truck on the way."

The latter endeavour is important, considering the context in which the information is garnered. Consider, for example, the process whereby the call-taker "interrogates" the caller (discussed further below). One of the call-taker's main goals is to elicit responses from the caller, mediated by the call-taker's cardset, to produce "evidence" in light of an interactional event between caller and call-taker that is far removed from traditional conceptions of evidence. Pre-hospital settings, for instance, are dissimilar to other emergency health contexts. Health care professionals at the hospital, for example, can rely on "objective" technologies (e.g., blood tests, ECG exams, devices to measure a patient's blood pressure, etc.) and senses of touch, vision, and smell to assess the patient. This is in contrast to the information collected and acted upon from the talk between call-taker and caller. This information – the evidence produced – is solely garnered from this verbal relational sequence between call-taker and caller.

As such, the EMD protocols are also aimed at minimizing, and theoretically eliminating, what call-takers, dispatchers, and managers at the Centre refer to as "freelancing" – a work practice that is considered a deviation from the EMD protocols, specifically when call-takers do not follow the protocols when speaking to callers (discussed in more detail below). The significance of eliminating freelance and encouraging call-takers to follow call-taking protocols was illustrated when managers at the Centre spoke about a quality assurance "sister process" associated with the EMD protocols. This sister process, as explained by a manager who helped implement it, is "a software package" that is embedded within a software program that allows data to be pulled from random calls "very objectively" so that calls can be evaluated and given quantified quality improvement scores, known as "QI score[s]." While the scores are important for quality improvement and quality assurance purposes, and for providing feedback to workers in the Centre, the Centre was also in the processes of becoming accredited; in order to become an accredited Centre, call-takers in the Centre had to maintain specific QI scores.

One manager who conducts these reviews explained that his assessments consist of listening to random recorded calls and using an evaluative schema provided by the accreditation body to assess different areas "that need to be met for accreditation." These assessment areas include, but are not limited to, 1) the case entry score, 2) the chief complaint, 3) the key questions, and 4) pre- and post-dispatch arrival instructions, which includes giving specific information or instructions to the caller based on the EMD protocol before and after an ambulance unit is dispatched. These areas are assessed, "each section gets a score," and a final score is determined that constitutes the "total compliance" of the call.

Another manager explained various reasons why call-takers would lose points based on the evaluative schema: 25 points are deducted if the address is not asked for or if it is not verified, 67 points if the call-taker identifies the wrong chief complaint/card, 33 points if the call-taker forgets to say, "OK, tell me exactly what happened" ("When you ask it that way, you're hoping that the caller will give you everything so that you can make a proper assessment of what's going on"). 10 points are deducted if questions are not asked in order, and 20 points if a call-taker freelances. One of the managers explained, "We're not allowed to freelance. You need to read these [key] questions verbatim is what they want to see." What counts for the reviewer, the Centre, and the accreditation body as it is organized by this review process is that certain sections for accreditation purposes have to have a score above 95 (e.g., case entry and chief complaint scores) while other sections need a score above 90 (e.g., key questions and pre- and post-dispatch instruction scores). Also important is the "overall score," which needs to be above 90. Another call-taker manager explained, "There's lots of review, specifically if a [call-taker] gets a score under 90; the report is being sent to the dispatch supervisor, the call evaluator supervisor, and we are following up with that employee."

This interchange between the call-taker and caller, as it is mediated by the EMD protocols, socially organizes this knowledge-production process, both for QI/QA purposes and as the information is transferred to dispatchers and paramedics on the streets; the work of the call-taker as she activates the EMD protocols is geared towards taming the dialogic interchange and producing evidence and evidence-based decision making in a context that lacks traditionally standard evidence. To further speed things up, and to increase the quality of evidence produced by the call-taker, a new system called ProQA was introduced in the Centre about a week after I began my observations, which essentially put the cardsets into a computer.

ProQA has a three-pronged focus: 1) to decrease the time it takes to process calls, 2) to increase the data collection and processing of the

Centre, and 3) to increase the compliance of call-takers. For example, ProQA supposedly "streamline(s) things" by taking the cardset out of the call-taker's hands; based on the information entered into the computer, "it automatically picks the determinant for you" (call-taker). A manager who played a role in implementing the technology explained that, in addition to freeing "up time so that you don't have to be looking from a cardset up to your screen," ProQA "provides us better recording data."

> It gives me a sequence of timestamps ... when did the call start, how long did it take me to do my key questions, how long did it take me to give my post-dispatch instructions, and some other timestamps. So, it gives us much more complete data than the cardset does, and that's valuable ... we can do things in ProQA that we cannot do in a cardset.

While decreasing the amount of time it takes to process calls and increasing the data-collection potential and, hence, facilitating better evaluation of calls by management, the introduction of ProQA was also intended to increase "compliance" and decrease the amount of "interpretation" and "freelancing" by call-takers; all of these measures are essential in order to become accredited. Because of ProQA, "our accreditation score" will increase (manager). As such, the focus of EMD as it is (re)emphasized by ProQA connects to discourses of risk and safety; risk is legally minimized when the cardset is followed. According to one call-taker, following the cardset "keeps you from getting into trouble, it keeps anyone from getting sued, because we can say oh, they were compliant in following protocol." Furthermore, when the cardset is followed, the correct resources are thought to be more efficiently deployed, representing more value for costs.

With the introduction of this technology, the work of evaluating calls has changed. One call-taker talked about having to "trust the system," as she was used to "knowing where I was going." With this said, she described the system as "good, it's really good ... It's kind of simplified a lot of things." As we will see later, call-takers activate these technologies and do interfacing work with their callers and the technologies to make the caller, the technologies, and ultimately their work "good."

Dispatchers – Alpha 1

As information is collected by the call-taker, it is entered into the computer and passed along to one of the two dispatchers. Known as Alpha 1 and Alpha 2, the dispatchers at the Centre have different responsibilities, as one manager of the Centre told me, to "control the fleet of about 50 to 52 units depending on the time of day." One dispatcher explained the demarcation of roles: Alpha 1 is primarily responsible for dispatching and flexing ambulance units and Alpha 2 provides support to the units after they are assigned to a call. More specifically, Alpha 1 has two primary roles. Their first role is to dispatch the "closest" unit; once the information from the call-taker "populates" Alpha 1's screen, the dispatcher hits "recommend" on the computer screen and the computer recommends the closest paramedic unit. The dispatcher then selects the unit and presses the "dispatch" button, and tones will be activated.

Alpha 1 is also responsible for ensuring that the crews in Calgary are managed effectively according to a deployment model known as "system status management" (SSM). This model, as one manager of dispatch explained, is geared towards facilitating the most efficient use of resources by ensuring that certain sections of the city are "covered" by ambulances. The model ensures "coverage" by applying "basic business principles of resource allocation, effectiveness and efficiency to EMS by utilizing historical data to accurately predict and allocate resources to fluctuating demands."[5] One dispatcher explained to me what he looks for in order to maintain coverage of the city:

> DISPATCHER: Yeah, I'm looking for any holes in the coverage. So, when I look at it I look to see OK, [Alpha 1] got the reds and the yellow covered, so [Alpha 1's] northwest looks pretty good.
> M: How do you know?
> DISPATCHER: I know because AHS has a deployment plan for metro where certain halls have to be covered, and what they've done is they've colour-coordinated them so the red halls are the most important ones, then your yellows, then your greens, and the way it works is what they're looking for is to have one of each colour covered in each district at all times … After 11:00 it kind of changes a little bit where you only have to have two of those colours covered, but then you're trying to make sure that that coverage is maintained. So, I know that, for example, this 34 is a red hall, so I know that it's covered. I know that she has a yellow covered in 31, so I know that she's maintaining her coverage.

This dispatcher is referring to the map of Calgary, which colour-codes the halls into red, yellow, and green, representing the priority of coverage respectively, a central feature of the deployment model. Depending on the "status" of crews in Calgary, paramedics might need to "flex" to different parts of the city in order to ensure "coverage." Red halls have to be covered (have an ambulance unit at the hall or nearby), whereas there is more flexibility in where ambulance units are stationed if they are assigned to a green hall.

According to Dan, the colour-coded status of a hall can have an impact on the amount of flexing a crew will do. Hanna and Dan and Jake and Julie, for example, were located at a green station. Because of this, they were "kind of in a bad spot" because they were one of the "flex trucks" in Calgary (Dan). I noticed during my ride-alongs that I would tend to flex more with Dan and Hanna and with Jake and Julie compared to other crews I rode with who were located at yellow or red colour-coded halls. Dan also explained that the colour of the station could impact the amount of downtime a crew would have, because "Dispatch will manoeuvre their resources around the city to make sure those [red] halls are covered." As a result, "some stations … when you come on, for a night shift, you kind of go and prepare your bed. Here it's just, if you got a few minutes to crash, then you do."

While Dan suggested that crews at red stations had more downtime, I observed the contrary. For example, the city centre crew, located at a red station, was probably the busiest crew I observed. While this might have been because I was observing them during a major event in Calgary, it also could have been because of their specialized mandate to treat and release "high-risk clientele." These observations can be contrasted with other crews I observed in the southwest city. These crews were located at a yellow station, which was where I experienced more downtime and the fewest calls compared to my other ride-alongs.

It is the responsibility of Alpha 1 to ensure that the city is covered, based on the deployment model. If there is a "hole" in the city, resources are supposed to be manoeuvred to ensure coverage. If resources are unavailable or limited – if certain "triggers" are met – then an alert system is activated: "if you have 11 or less [units available for a call] you call a yellow alert. Once you hit 8 you're in an orange [alert] … and then a red alert is none. Reds are bad" (call-taker manager). The work of the dispatch manager also orients to the deployment of resources and the work of Alpha 1. In addition to keeping track of the number of units available for a call (green units) and monitoring the work of Alpha 1 to ensure appropriate coverage in the city, it is this manager who activates the alert system once these triggers are met.

Once an alert is activated, all EMS units, including their managers and emergency department staff, are informed. A dispatch manager explained that when the city is in an alert, EDs are "supposed to try and release one ambulance [at the hospital] ... within 10 minutes and then one additional ambulance from each hospital every 20 minutes for the duration of the alert." The EMS supervisor's work is coordinated by these alerts, which further coordinates the work of paramedics. One EMS supervisor explained how being in alert impacts him and his crews:

> It depends on what platoon you're on. If you're on one of the platoons that has the more micro-managey type managers, then, and I ... didn't really like it, then they'll [EMS supervisor] kinda start breathing down everybody's neck, crawling all over everybody, you know, "Clear up, double up, roar roar roar." We're a little more casual about it here on this platoon. Normally it sorts itself out. Occasionally, like if you start getting really low on trucks, you know down to five trucks, so then you'll see supes start busting to the hospital to, "Hey ... guys, out."

A manager with AHS who works in the Centre explained that when the system is in alert, part of his work is to ensure that EMS supervisors go "out there" to the hospital and ask, "Who can leave, who can go now, and the hospitals are usually pretty good again at downloading these patients off ... " He went on to explain that solving the problem of "hitting alerts" is accomplished through "effectively ... managing" the system by essentially "kick[ing]" paramedics out who are "hang[ing] around the hospital," which puts additional pressure on the hospitals to take in EMS patients.

Dispatchers – Alpha 2

When paramedics "are assigned" a call, they switch their radios to Alpha 2, known as the "working channel." Alpha 2 is responsible for maintaining contact with the unit after it is dispatched to a call by checking in every 15 minutes to ensure that the crew is safe. Paramedics acknowledge that they are safe by saying, "Code 15." In addition to maintaining contact with all the units on a call in Calgary, the work of Alpha 2 is to "give [paramedics] anything they need," including "manpower," like medical backup, police, or fire, and to answer "any questions that they have," like the location of the patient.

One dispatcher described his work as Alpha 2 as "not even dispatching paramedics, but as management of resources." In addition, a central part of the work that Alpha 2 does is to track paramedics' time, which makes up a key performance measure of the EMS system. Tracked times for paramedics include the time it takes for them to leave for the scene once dispatched, when they arrive at the scene, when they depart from the scene, when they arrive at the hospital, and when they depart from the hospital and are ready for another call.

It is also important to note that the call-taker will sometimes remain on the phone with the caller after the call is transferred to the dispatchers, sometimes even until the ambulance arrives. The goal is for the call-taker to collect additional "pertinent" information from the caller, which will then be entered into the computer and transferred to the paramedics on the streets. This was illustrated in the previous chapters when the paramedic in the passenger seat would orient to the CAD as it was updated on the way to a call. Furthermore, with the caller still on the phone with the call-taker, the dispatcher might, for example, stand up and ask the call-taker a question or phone them, based on questions posed by the street paramedics to the dispatcher.

The work of Alpha 2 interfaces with the Regional Emergency Patient Access and Coordination system (REPAC). REPAC is a technology that analyses information from the Regional Emergency Department Information Systems (REDIS) and synthesizes it into "virtually real-time information" about emergency department capacity (McLeod et al., 2010, p. 1384).[6] What results are colour-coded status indicators of different hospitals in Calgary: green, yellow, orange, and red. If a hospital reaches a certain "trigger" determined (and changeable) by upper-level managers/administrators, the colour status of the hospital changes, which "relates to acuity, volumes, you know, if things are backing up in the department, etc." (manager).

Prior to the introduction of REPAC, as one paramedic explained, the hospital that paramedics would go to was based on factors like "preference," the location of the call – "We're in the south, well, let's go to D5 [the code of one of the hospitals in Calgary]" – and information received from dispatch, whereby "dispatch would occasionally warn you and say, 'Hey look, there's eight trucks at D5, you might not want to go there.' 'Oh, OK,' so you'd go somewhere else." With the compiled information produced by and through REPAC, paramedics now ask dispatch for "REPAC please." Alpha 2 then looks at her REPAC screen, located next to her other screens, and checks the status of hospitals – the status "determine[s] priority" (manager of dispatch). Alpha 2 then relays the information to the paramedics about the "top" choices of hospitals in Calgary to transport patients to.

REPAC was described by one of the managers who helped implement it as a "guide" for paramedics in their decision making. Furthermore, there are certain situations that can "override" REPAC, such as if EMS is in red alert or if the patient meets certain "destination criteria" – for example, the patient is having a stroke or is in need of immediate resuscitation. If a paramedic decides to override REPAC, an EMS supervisor explained to me, "technically you're supposed to write a risk management every time you override the REPAC destination. Nobody does it, and some people just don't follow REPAC. It's not enforced really."

While most of the paramedics I observed would take the patient to the hospital that the patient requested, whether it was the hospital they were REPACed to or not, this was not always the case. During one observation with Carl, an EMT-P with over 20 years of experience, and Russ, an EMT with less than five years of experience, I noticed this sequence of events as they were loading an older patient into the ambulance: Carl turns and tilts his head to the side, puts his hand to his walkie-talkie, presses the button on its side, and says, "REPAC please." Dispatch responds, "D7," which is the hospital across town. With his hand off the walkie-talkie, Carl responds, "Ouch." Russ also responds in a sarcastic tone, "That's close." After the patient is loaded into the ambulance, Russ contacts the Dispatch Centre and asks for REPAC again. Dispatch replies again with "D7." Russ then mentions to Carl that the patient's wife wants the hospital located in their neighbourhood. Carl shakes his head, and Russ responds, "Not happening." An interchange between the patient and Carl follows. The patient asks Carl, "Are we going to [the hospital of the patient's preference]?" Carl responds in a stern voice, "No," and explains to the patient that they will be going to the hospital on the other side of the city. The patient replies, "Oh no, why is that?" Carl responds, "It is the fastest way to see the doctor ... I wish we could go to [the closer hospital], but they are very busy." With the patient looking disappointed, we leave for D7.

Even though REPAC was "not really enforced," based on my observations with paramedics on the streets, REPAC was compelling in that those whom I observed used the technology frequently, even if it did not reflect the preferences of the paramedics in terms of which hospital they liked going to or the wishes of their patients. Russ, for example, explained after the aforementioned call that the hospital the patient wanted to go to was in "red" and that it made "no sense to take him there and wait all night."

In the age of technological governance, the REPAC technology is intended to lessen the diversions of ambulances away from hospitals that do not currently have the capacity to accept them because of a lack of resources (McLeod et al., 2010, p. 1384). By directing crews to hospitals that have capacity, the technology is institutionally viewed as being "effective" in that it results "in the more efficient and rational provision of emergency services and may mitigate the effects of ED crowding on ambulance diversions" (p. 1384) and thus creates "a balance between supply and capacity" (p. 1387). In this sense, REPAC connects to the admission, discharge, and transfer (ADT) system discussed by Rankin and Campbell (2006) in that REPAC is geared towards "tam[ing] the movement of" (p. 45) ambulances and the work of paramedics and supporting "the movement of patients in, through the system, and out of hospital beds, expeditiously, on the basis of information that relates these activities to costs" (p. 46). The goal is to manage resources as efficiently and effectively as possible:

> A hospital can only achieve maximum possible efficiency when fixed investments are fully utilized ... If capacity under-utilization exists, fixed costs are higher than necessary and average resource costs of treatment are not being minimized. Therefore, while some degree of spare capacity is essential to meet periods of peak demand ... excessive spare capacity generates inefficiency and needs to be identified. (Kerr et al., 1999, p. 640, cited in Rankin & Campbell, 2006, p. 45)

The coordinative power of this technology is its ability to organize, direct, and even "predict" the need for services. The manager of REPAC explained that this is not just "predictive" in its ability to "absorb the load of EMS transports" (McLeod et al., 2010, p. 1384) but can also be used to determine "if we need additional physicians [in the hospital] to be able to ... get us back into green status ... We're predicting ... We're telling you you're starting to get into trouble" (REPAC manager).

On the Centre's Floor – Interfacing or Discretionary Work

... the European navigator begins with a plan – a course – which he has charted according to certain universal principles, and he carries out his voyage by relating his every move to that plan. His effort throughout his voyage is directed to remaining "on course." If unexpected events occur he must first alter the plan, then respond accordingly. The Trukese navigator begins with an objective rather than a plan. He sets off toward the objective and responds to conditions as they arise in an ad hoc fashion. He utilizes information provided by the wind, the waves, the tide and current, the fauna, the stars, the clouds, the sound of the water on the side of the boat, and he steers accordingly. His effort is directed to doing whatever is necessary to reach the objective. If asked, he can point to his objective at any moment, but he cannot describe his course.

(Berreman, 1966, p. 347, cited in Suchman, 2007, p. 24)

While the work described in the previous section suggests that the roles of Alpha 1 and Alpha 2 are separate, in practice there is much interplay between the two dispatchers as well as between the dispatchers and the call-takers. As such, the work described in the previous sections should not be thought of as being completely separate or sequential; call-takers orient to the work of dispatchers, who also orient to the work of call-takers. For instance, information that is processed from the call-takers continuously "updates" the dispatchers. As information is sent to the dispatchers, dispatchers also "filter" through the call-taker information. According to one call-taker, call-takers and dispatchers try to "work as a cohesive unit, as a team, and get, you know, the right address down so that, you know, we do this consistently making the best use of our resources." Similarly, one dispatcher described how she constantly listens and orients to the work of the other dispatcher "to make sure everything's OK ... We try to be just one step ahead ... Because you'll think you have it all under control and then you'll start losing [coverage in Calgary] ... Then I have to start pulling trucks [to cover]."

The work described above is a simplified version of what actually happens on the Centre's floor. This simplified version suggests that there is little, if any, discretion in accomplishing the work of dispatchers and call-takers (Pence, 2001). In fact, and as alluded to above, limiting discretion and increasing compliance are major tasks of the technologies central to the work of dispatchers and call-takers. However, in between the official and simplified versions of tasks on the one hand and the accounting of those tasks on the other is what might be thought of as discretionary or *interfacing work*. McCoy (personal communication, 2013) describes interfacing work as follows:

All front-line people do interface work – between particular individuals/ situations and an institutional work process/documentary order.

Sometimes they have to do a lot of work in order to create a for-the-purposes satisfactory or workable fit. This takes skill. It is essential to the work of the agency, to the deployment of any standardized protocol. People who know about the work generally know – take for granted – that this work is being done, even if it is not made visible in the official version.[7]

There is much work that goes into trying to make callers "good," as expressed in a mantra I heard throughout my time at the Centre: "You're only as good as your caller." More generally, there is much interfacing work that goes into accomplishing the official tasks of people in the Centre. This was exemplified when paramedics spoke about "the good ones" (Jake) in reference to certain call-takers and dispatchers. I will next focus on some of this interfacing work of call-takers and then move on to a discussion of the interfacing work of dispatchers.

Such interfacing work becomes more visible when calls do not go as planned. There is unrecorded work that accomplishes the official documentation process, such as the work of trying to calm the caller down and to elicit talk from the caller.

Call-taker: [*Phone rings*] 911, for what city? [*Pause*] And do you need police, fire, or ambulance? [*Pause*] OK, what's going on? [*Long pause*] OK, OK, lis–, hello? OK, listen. You need to tell me where you are please. [*Pause*] OK, 12th station like as in 12th Street? Bus station? [*Pause*] OK, ma'am, hello? Hello? Hi, I need you to talk to me, OK? Don't talk to her for a minute, I need you to talk to me. What's the [*pause*] OK, well I need you to talk to me. You called 911, I need you to talk to me. And you said … ? [*Pause. Sounds of call-taker typing in the background*] OK, well is anybody else there that's [from Calgary] that can [*inaudible*]? [*Pause*] OK. What's the phone num– ? [*Long pause*] She's saying that she's across the street from the 12th Street bus station, is that right? OK. Can you tell me what's happening there? [*Pause*] OK. [*Pause*] At her knee? [*Sounds of call-taker typing in the background*] OK. You can put her on the phone now, thanks. [*Pause*] Hello? Hello? Hello? Hi. Hi, is [*pause*] OK. Lis– , hello? Hello? No, you're not going to hang up on me. You can't hang up on me. Are you going to talk to me? [*The caller hangs up*] Oh my fucking god.

Calls do not always go as planned. In the example above, the call-taker has difficulty getting the caller to listen and respond to her questions. One call-taker, who had many years of experience, explained that "one of the most important things I was taught when I originally did my EMD training ... was repetitive persistence, so an action and a result – I need you to calm down so we can help your daughter." This call-taker also explained that she was taught to "stop talking" when callers are not calm. Other call-takers talked about the need to provide "positive reassurance" when dealing with a caller who is "freaking out" – "No ma'am, you have to calm yourself and we have to do what we can do now to help your husband ... you're doing a good job, keep it up ..." Such work can be thought of as *the work of making a good caller*. In essence, as one call-taker described it, there is "lots of grey area" when it comes to working with callers. She explained that "some callers are way better than others. Some answer the questions significantly better than others, and sometimes it's you know ... You're panicked or something ... There are people who just don't listen ... You're only as good as your caller."[8]

Even calls that are relatively straightforward require interfacing work that makes a caller good. Call-takers, for example, attempt to elicit answers that are commensurable with the dispatch cardset by rephrasing the question or using "different language," or asking the question in a "different way." Adding to the complexity of the work is that callers are also not standard. One call-taker talked about "chatty" people and how sometimes, as a call-taker, you need to "hurry them along" because "I need to know right now that he's having chest pain, and he's clammy, and that he needs a Delta response." Another call-taker described the opposite with chatty people, explaining that, rather than hurrying callers along, she tends to "let people talk," and she listens for answers from the caller "before I ask the questions." While this call-taker has a "hard time interrupting older people now," if she needs more "information" on something that the caller says, "I'll kind of cut in and ask the questions."

While hurrying callers or "cut[ting] in and ask[ing] questions" is important because time is of the essence in emergency medical situations, call-takers also orient to their work contexts. This became visible to me when call-takers oriented to the light flashing at the top of their terminals, which is an indication that callers are waiting in the "queue." One call-taker explained that when this happens, she tries to "wrap up my call" by "quickly" giving instructions to the caller, essentially speeding things up. Furthermore, call-takers might orient to this context – "if the light's flashing" – when they are not on a call, in a sense activating the significance of lights flashing, either by "hurry[ing] up" when they are on a break to get back to their terminal or avoiding going to the bathroom or on break "until it slows down a bit."

Calls do not always go according to how they are envisioned in the cardset because callers and their contexts are not standard. Therefore, there is complex work involved with trying to organize the talk into a chief complaint. Such complexity is contrary to what the cardset suggests because it is assumed in the protocols that a chief complaint can be identified if call-takers are "compliant" in reading the cards. This simplistic conceptualization of the interchange between caller and call-taker was reflected in, and simultaneously critiqued by, one participant who talked about the challenges of identifying a chief complaint vis-à-vis key questions.

> Call-taker: ... "OK, tell me exactly what happened." Just that sentence alone will let the caller give you the exact story of what actually happened ... If somebody says oh, somebody's bleeding from their nose, that could easily be a card 21 for hemorrhage for a nosebleed, right? ... But the question where it actually asks, "OK, tell me exactly what happened?" "Oh, well he fell off a ladder and he hit his head and now he's bleeding from his nose." That changes the whole situation, right? So, just asking that one question ... It's now a fall instead of a 21 hemorrhage. What's the difference? The questions, right? ... Sometimes you do start to question yourself; "Oh, am I on the right chief complaint ... Is this a stroke or is it really a chest pain?" ... but again as long as you're able to follow the protocol you shouldn't be able to have that [*inaudible*]. I mean nothing in this dispatch environment is black and white. I think sometimes it is a grey ...

Call-takers also discussed this in relation to ProQA. One said, "Technically, if I ask any questions outside of the protocols, I'm freelancing and I can lose points. So, do you do it sometimes? Yeah, you do, because you're clarifying what that person said, but technically you're supposed to read it exactly how it's written, right." Another call-taker said, "Sometimes I think it's silly and I try and be compliant, I really do, I really try, but sometimes the questions don't make any sense for the situation ... Like I know it's supposed to eliminate any error ... I love ProQA but at the same time, I don't know how much you can put human behaviour into a computer system." This call-taker was referring to the context of the call and how there is not always a standard "flow":

It depends how the call's flowing. If the call's flowing really easy, it's easy to stick to ProQA, but if they throw you a curveball, like "Not really," or "I don't know," it's more like this, yeah, and then I find myself clarifying a lot more.

Much of this interfacing work became visible when the call-takers talked about how they record and pass along the information they collect from the callers to different people; some information is entered into the computer and passed along to dispatchers for data collection purposes, categorizing the call, and allocation of resources (some of this information appears on the CADs in the ambulance unit), and some of the information is entered into the computer for use by paramedics on the streets because some information is "relevant, even though it's not at all in the cards" (call-taker).

Information that is not in the cards is entered into the computer as "remarks" or "notes" and appears on the CAD screen in the ambulance unit, sometimes in all capital letters so it is easily identified by paramedics on the streets. This information gives paramedics "an idea" of what to expect – "to sort of give the medics sort of a better picture of everything" – such as "underlying medical issues" or scene safety issues that might impact their work. One call-taker explained that entering notes is not something "you need to do, but I think once you've dispatched and … [know] what they're looking for … then …" Another call-taker explained that the information entered into this section is "not per protocol" but rather based on the experience of knowing what paramedics might need, like the clothes people are wearing, specific location details, what the patient looks like, including "ethnicity, as well as their height, hair colour," type of vehicle they are looking for, if they need to gain access to an apartment, the code to open the door. It was this information in the remarks section that many of the paramedics I spoke with relied on the most.

Such discretionary or interfacing work does not stop with call-takers; there is also much work that goes into accomplishing the tasks of dispatching, whether it is the anticipatory work of successfully implementing the deployment model in Calgary or the seemingly simple act of pressing a button when the "closest" unit has been identified. For example, dispatching the closest unit via the "recommend" button is not so clear-cut, because while one unit might be geographically closer, the unit might be going "southbound … and can't get turned around faster than a unit that's a little bit further away." Knowing the geographic locale of where paramedics work comes into play for dispatchers and can be essential in dispatching the unit that is actually closer in terms of response time than geographic distance, even though it appears further away according to the computer technology.

Discretionary work for Alpha 1 is also invoked in relation to the alert system in Calgary. This includes a lot of "juggling" work that occurs in order to prevent alerts from happening or to prevent them from getting worse. This work inevitably interfaces with the "downtime" of paramedics in terms of flexing. One individual explained this from two overlapping perspectives, as she was not only an acting manager of dispatchers but also a dispatcher.

> From a dispatcher perspective it requires, you know … it's this constant vigilance. So, what you're doing, it's constantly looking at your screen, seeing, paging people, you're doing a lot more flexing [when alerts are "hit"] trying to get your areas covered, because you might have lost an entire area of the city, but still have four down south, you know, so you're moving trucks to be able to cover the areas that you need to cover. So, right now [referring to the current dispatcher on duty] she's got three trucks in [one section]. She doesn't need three trucks [there] … she needs to page one of them out to come into [the city centre].

Similarly, another dispatcher talked about the work of flexing as a "game of chess." Pointing to her screen as I was observing her work, she explained it like this:

> Also you have the option of having a red and a green, because you always have to [have] a red covered, it can be any of the reds. So, it could be this hall and this hall, and for this time at 1:00 am, it can be this hall and this hall, or it can be this hall and this hall, or it can be this hall and this hall, right? So, but if you have like 34 covered and 17 covered, then you have a big, again, gaping hole in the middle.

Context matters and will impact how a dispatcher actually activates and accomplishes the deployment plan. The same dispatcher explained the importance of context:

> You get a long weekend and you just get hammered, and hammered, and hammered in the [downtown] core. I'm OK to take this truck and cover the core a little bit more … so that maybe something big will happen, at least I have that truck there, right? So, but during the daytime it is a little

bit different … always have to have your red halls covered, but if you have a red and a green, you don't have to have your yellow covered again …

Another dispatcher said, "It's like a chess game you never win." This individual explained that coverage of the city sometimes gets "ugly" with not enough vehicles. When this happens, this dispatcher starts worrying and "crossing her fingers" and begins to "deploy" certain resources that she would otherwise not deploy, like EMS managers or specialty teams that are supposed to be used for specific emergent purposes; for example, the city centre team that specializes in treating "high-risk clientele" might be shifted to a different part of Calgary.

Other dispatchers spoke about "manipulating," "bend[ing]," or "stretching" the rules – "We can't break them," one dispatcher adamantly said. For example, one dispatcher explained how she does not always send "the closest unit" to low-priority (Alpha) calls. This dispatcher said that she does this to facilitate crew change, described by some dispatchers as a challenging part of the job, and to "cut back on the overtime." The level of priority (e.g., Alpha) of a call gives dispatchers "a little bit of latitude on who we can send." Dispatchers also spoke about "protecting" paramedics when they are doing a "pick up," code name for having coffee, lunch, or taking a break. To do so, they will put another unit on if it is a low-priority call.

According to one dispatcher, "Every single function has their own SOPs [standard operating procedures] … They're the rules and guidelines that we are bound by as call-takers, as dispatchers … and all the [frequent protocol] updates that we get are to go hand-in-hand with what AHS wants and expects." Characteristic of interfacing work is providing a "social perspective" to the highly organized site of the Centre, where the smooth functioning of the system is not simply achieved by being "compliant" or simply following the rules; there is an artful interplay between the workplace as an institutional setting and what happens on the ground of that setting. One dispatcher described this interplay between dispatchers, paramedics, and SOPs as a "bit of a game of accommodating" or of staying as "close" as possible to the "operating procedures" while not treating paramedics as "robots."

Discussion and Conclusion

The work of evaluating calls and dispatching ambulance services is a highly coordinated, text-mediated process that inevitably interfaces with and organizes the work of paramedics on the streets. This chapter extended our look at the work of paramedics by focusing on how their work connects to and is socially organized by people who work at the Dispatch Centre in Calgary. I provided an in-depth examination of the complex work of people in the Centre and focused specifically on how their work interfaced with and was organized by others vis-à-vis different institutional technologies.

The institutional ethnographic focus here moved beyond a focus on "naturally" occurring talk in a Dispatch Centre and examined how people's work in the Centre, and their talk, are socially organized; what people in the Centre do – their actual work processes – interfaces with and is made interfaceable to the institutional settings, technologies central to their work settings, and regimes of accountability. I also exemplified how the talk between callers and call-takers is not just coordinated between each other but, at least in the 21st century, is also a product of coordinated social relational sequences where call-takers draw their callers into text-mediated work processes in order to accomplish successful call taking and sufficient "evidence" that institutionally reflects "quality." Also, by focusing on the interfacing work that is done by Alpha 1 and Alpha 2 in terms of dispatching and managing EMS resources in Calgary, this chapter provided an in-depth examination of emergency medical call taking and dispatching work in contemporary society.

The interfacing technologies that I focused on in this chapter include the EMD protocols and the newly introduced ProQA system, the SSM deployment model, and REPAC. In addition to helping accomplish the work of people in the Centre and paramedics on the streets, these technologies are geared towards creating and producing efficiencies and using resources in the "best" and most "appropriate" way. For example, key to the work of Alpha 1 in flexing and activating the alert system, and to the work of Alpha 2 in sending paramedics to the most appropriate hospital, is a "downloading" of work processes onto paramedics (e.g., doubling up, transporting patients to hospital outside of their location of comfort, and EMS supervisors "breathing down everybody's neck" to get paramedics out of the hospital more quickly), front-line workers in the hospital (e.g., nurses [see Melon, 2012]), and even the patient and the patient's family (e.g., patients being brought to a hospital far from their place of residence and social support system). Hidden dangers can result from these text-mediated practices, such as the rapport between paramedics and nurses being eroded as paramedics go to hospitals that they might otherwise not go to, patients being transported to hospitals far from where their friends and family live (see chapter 2), or emergency departments being "slammed." According to one nurse I spoke with:

> They'll send 10 ambulances to [one hospital] because [it is] in green, well then that puts you in red ... That system, REPAC ... that system doesn't seem to work very well, and I mean that'll happen at [other hospitals] too; they'll send us like four in a row and we'll go why are you sending them here ... you just kind of watch and go oh my gosh, like how can you do this? ... Like come on, so yeah ... a big tension with REPAC.

An acting paramedic supervisor, Dave, expressed similar sentiments:

> What just about kills me is that they send us here when it's like this, when we're just going to go straight to the hall. That's just absolutely asinine. The whole idea of this REPAC system ... It used to be that you just picked wherever you wanted to go, so now you have to call and ask for a REPAC ... We were told that the REPAC destinations available to us when we left [for the hospital] were both green. So [*pause*] we come here, oh it's a green hospital and we get punted to the bloody hall ... The whole claim with this thing was that it was gonna reduce that ... from what I've been privy to in my position, it hasn't helped EMS out at all, in fact it's kind of hurt us a bit. But supposedly the higher uppers like it so it stays. The hospital staff don't seem to like it either 'cause what happens is each hospital in succession ends up getting slammed with, you know, tag teamed with ambulances ... it's like a dog pile with each hospital.

Irrespective of the consequences, it is through this downloading of work that efficiencies are garnered through targeting front-line work and expanding resources already deployed through technological coordination and control. As one manager explained of the current reform, there has been a renewed focus on "are the SOPs being followed, are the cars getting there on time, are we moving cars around to cover the areas properly ... " The unwritten mantra that is guiding governance on the front line of EMS is doing more with less or at least with the same amount of resources – "Have we checked all the cars at the hospital, and have patients been doubled up at the hospital, and what's causing our alert?" (manager)

While these technologies structure and organize the work of front-line workers, this chapter also showed that there is an artful interplay between how these technologies are theoretically conceptualized and how they are used in practice; there is much discretionary or interfacing work that goes on in the Centre to counteract the limitations of the technologies and ensure that the complexities of front-line work are reflected in the technologies via their work processes. Furthermore, many of the work processes of call-takers and dispatchers and their work orientation to the here and now of the contingencies of their work setting are cut out from the information produced by the technologies embedded within this work setting. The institutional technologies central to this work setting make visible only snippets of actual work practices, based on "objective" information required to move the information on to other processing interchanges.

What results from, and ultimately reproduces, this social organization of knowledge are ideological practices of (not) knowing, whereby information is provided in objectified form (e.g., performance scores of call-takers, accreditation scores, etc.), and this is part of how the information is a priori conceptualized (Rankin & Campbell, 2006, p. 128; see also Smith, 1990). Porter (1995) discusses the use of public statistics in this context. He writes, "Public statistics are able to describe social reality partly because they help to define it ... the quantitative technologies used to investigate social and economic life work best if the world they aim to describe can be remade in their image" (p. 43). Similarly, the official account of the effectiveness of REPAC is that it is "effective" in managing and "mitigate[ing] the effects of ED crowding on ambulance diversions" (McLeod et al., 2010, p. 1384). The work of dealing with and accomplishing the efficiencies is left outside the official account of what is happening, along with the consequences. What results is a disjuncture between the official account of REPAC and how its consequences take shape in practice, as exemplified in the quotation at the beginning of this chapter.

The reporting of actual work is a simplistic abstraction of that work, geared towards standardizing patients, the work of paramedics, and the knowledge they produce. For example, the "Monthly Emergency Medical Services Activity Summary" reports key performance indicators, including *Response Times* – "the time elapsed from when a call is received at an EMS dispatch centre until the first EMS unit arrives on scene" – and *Events Volume* – the "number of individual events that EMS responded to." Response times are measured for "life-threatening events," classified as Delta or Echo calls, and the volume of events is categorized into "emergency events" and "non-emergency events," with the former being defined by calls that are classified as Bravo, Charlie, Delta, and Echo calls.[9]

This standardized view of work and "objective" information produced by and through the technologies is often contrary to the work orientation of paramedics on the streets and the people who work in the Dispatch Centre. For example, in addition to the objective information passed from the Centre to paramedics via the CAD, paramedics also orient to the subjective "notes" produced by call-takers, information that represents the non-standard aspects of the call. This disjuncture between information produced objectively and information produced subjectively was exemplified and came to the fore when many of the paramedics I spoke with called into question the information they received from the Centre. This questioning of information did not seem to be about the veracity of the information produced, but rather about the type of information passed on. Whereas the call type mattered for call-takers in terms of how their work was evaluated, what counted for paramedics on the streets were primarily the "notes." With the introduction of ProQA, the amount of information paramedics received on their CAD significantly increased. While a manager at the Centre said that ProQA provides the crews with "much better information than they ever [had] before and that's key," I asked one paramedic to speak about the new and "better information" they now receive. He immediately responded, "I hate it. I hate the new notes. I like the old notes." He explained the difference between the old and new notes and how his work has changed as a result:

> Just doesn't read as well. You used to just get the notes, the pertinents, now it's got like names and QA [quality assurance] blah, blah, blah, and it's all this extraneous bullshit that we don't need. We get all the notes that the call-taker's taking instead of the ones we really need. Like I don't care what her name is and that she's gonna call her dad. Like I want to know, is this guy breathing, puking, chest pain. Is he fighting? You know does he have a weapon? That's the stuff I want to know. Now I'm constantly doing this [searching through the notes] ... I'm going to miss stuff ... like hold-backs 'cause there's so many notes now you can miss, like OK he's got a gun that they've missed, and now you'll walk into a bad scene. Sometimes more information isn't good.

As such, the knowledge collected from the Centre, codified into call types, and passed on to the EMS crews reflected a paradigmatic understanding of knowledge geared towards objective management and better resource allocation that does not always jibe with the ongoing, unfolding reality of what paramedics experience on the streets. For example, holdbacks are activated when concerns for paramedics' safety are suspected; if a call-taker hears fighting in the background or suspects something suspicious while talking on the phone with an individual, for instance, they will place a holdback on the call. Dispatch will notify paramedics via the CAD that a holdback is in place, and the paramedic unit will wait at a safe location not too far away from the scene until police are able to confirm that it is safe for the paramedics to attend. Sometimes holdbacks are missed or placed too late on the call, which can jeopardize the safety of paramedics because crews might go to the scene rather than wait. Furthermore, after ProQA was introduced, I observed a dispatcher at work at the Centre who explained to me that a crew had missed a holdback. The dispatcher explained that "we tried our best" to update the crew. She then went on to say, "They have this new system now though, unfortunately, and all of this is given to them [*referring to information on her screen*], and it's a lot of information for them to read. They're used to seeing this part only [*pointing to a smaller amount of information on the screen*]." The dispatcher then explained that it was "their [paramedics'] due diligence to read that call."

This analysis brings the artfulness of the work of actually accomplishing the official tasks of people in the Dispatch Centre to light and confronts a system that is being organized by technologies that produce information based on a positivist view of people, their work, and language, akin to the European navigator trope of Berremans quoted in the epigraph of section 6.5. The interfacing work of call-takers in codifying talk and trying to elicit "appropriate" talk from callers, the organizing and coordinating of dispatchers, and the orienting work of paramedics with the information produced by the Centre are all socially organized into a one-dimensional view of objective-objectified happenings. In other words, the everyday work practices described here and illustrated and emphasized in the Trukese navigator trope – "Although the objective of the Trukese navigator is clear from the outset, his actual course is contingent on unique circumstances that he cannot anticipate[10] in advance" (Suchman, 2007, p. 25) – are processed and quantified with the assumption that effective management of workers will meet the system's needs. My goal in this chapter was to begin to describe and explicate these work processes.

Objectified views of work and the demarcation of institutional accounts of happenings and the resulting "objective" knowledge that is processed through the organizing discourse assume that maximal efficiency of the system can be reached through effective governance of resources and workers. This chapter brings to light some disjunctures and alludes to some of the consequences of such text-mediated practices. Furthermore, what became clear through this analysis, and what is analytically interesting, is the work involved in call-takers drawing callers into their work processes, the work that Alpha 1 and Alpha 2 do as they work with and work on the technologies that interface with dispatching paramedics on the street, and how the information the technologies collect is put together into institutionally recognized forms of knowledge, primarily in the form of time (e.g., response times) and acuity of calls (e.g., Alpha, Bravo, Charlie, Delta, and Echo). This institutionally produced and recognized knowledge is not what counts for paramedics and is not the only information that counts for workers in the Centre.

In exploring the interfacing and discretionary work that is central to the success of the Centre, this investigation ethnographically brings to light what is otherwise cut out yet inseparable from the "validity" produced by and through institutional technologies at the Centre. By providing empirical evidence that is grounded in the actual work of people and by showing how reforms are playing out in practice, I explicate how the work of paramedics connects to, and is organized by, governance practices off the streets. The next chapter continues this line of analysis by further exploring how the work of paramedics is organized and coordinated and how knowledge of that work becomes visible in the age of technological governance.

Chapter Seven

Taming and Creating Knowledge of Front-Line Work

Introduction

Emergencies are unplanned. Hence, the work of paramedics and other front-line workers is by definition uncertain. The nature of uncertain work complicates the implementation of the new public management strategies that "re-conceiv[e] and, to some extent reorganiz[e], many if not all organizational activities (support and administration as well as production or service) as work processes involving identifiable inputs, outputs and customers" (McCoy, 1991, p. 9, cited in Rankin & Campbell, 2006, p. 45). As a result, there is much text-mediated social organization that goes into making the work of paramedics visible and governable.

The previous chapter took readers behind the scenes of emergency services and into the Dispatch Centre. We saw different institutional technologies activated by people at work; these technologies entered into and organized some of the work processes of paramedics on the streets. This chapter extends our look into the social organization of emergency medical services by further exploring the interfacing technologies that were introduced in chapters 2 through 4. I focus specifically on two technologies, the Medical Control Protocols (hereafter protocols), which are geared towards targeting and taming clinical practices, and the electronic Patient Care Record (ePCR), a technological device capturing institutionally relevant information that, along with other text-mediated information, plays an integral role in quality improvement and quality assurance projects that are increasingly targeting front-line EMS work.

The targeting of work and the production of "valid" data, as facilitated by and through the institutional technologies discussed here and in the last chapter, must be considered within the context of the current reform practices in pre-hospital emergency settings. This need to produce valid data is highlighted in a review by the Health Quality Council of Alberta entitled "Review of Operations of Ground Emergency Medical Services in Alberta" (hereafter the Review). The Review stated that there are concerns "about the availability and adequacy of EMS data at a provincial level to effectively measure and manage the performance of the EMS system" (Health Quality Council of Alberta [HQCA], 2013, p. 3). In fact, the Review highlighted the benefits of centralizing the provincial EMS system and, by proxy, having a standardized set of provincial protocols: "(1) evidence-based care, medical oversight and auditing can be standardized; (2) resources can be more efficiently and effectively managed; and (3) data can be better managed, reported on, and used to support quality management" (p. 4). From the vantage point of Alberta Health Services (AHS), centralization of emergency medical services can be seen as better facilitating the instillation of quality improvement and assurance "culture" (pp. 236–7).

It is important to note that, while this chapter is separate from chapter 6, the technologies examined here interface with the institutional technologies discussed in that chapter; both sets of technologies play a role in the managerial agenda, which is an integral thread throughout this analysis. As such, this chapter should be viewed as complementing chapter 6; whereas chapter 6 explored technologies that target the efficient allocation of emergency medical space (REPAC) and "labour resources" (EMD protocols, ProQA, and the deployment model) (Rankin & Campbell, 2006, p. 85), this chapter explores technologies of knowledge and governance that are targeting clinical practice (protocols) and knowledge production practices central to accountability and quality improvement projects (ePCR) in EMS. While there are distinctions between the aspects of work practices and institutional settings these technologies target, I suggest that the technologies blend together in the project of producing institutional, text-mediated representations of work geared towards reforming the work of front-line workers and the health care system.

Following this introduction, the chapter is organized into five sections, followed by a discussion and conclusion. The next section provides a brief look into the historical developments that led to the wide use of protocols in health care and pre-hospital emergency medical services. In the third section, I discuss the ePCR as a technology that was introduced for a multiplicity of purposes aligned with the agenda of reforming pre-hospital emergency settings, such as to increase compliance with protocols and produce text-mediated knowledge of that compliance, to improve data collection and processing practices, and to facilitate the efficient use of EMS resources. In the fourth section, I discuss the work of different players behind the scenes who intersect with the ePCR, the protocols, and standardized texts used for assessment and evaluative purposes in order to ensure that paramedics comply with these technologies and provide "good" care. In this analysis, we see the work that goes into the socially organized production of compliance (McCoy, 2009). In the fifth section, I discuss the potential of the ePCR as a "business intelligence tool" that is being used to organize and reorganize the work of paramedics based on snippets of institutionally relevant information collected from the ePCR and other data sources. In the sixth section, I trace relations of governance and accountability by providing readers with three figures that depict the social organization of knowledge in EMS in Calgary and elsewhere.

Protocols and the Targeting of Clinical Practice

According to Chappell, McDonald, and Stones (2008), the era of accountability, coordination, and control characteristic of contemporary health care emerged during the "discontent" of the 1980s and the 1990s (p. 398). During this time period, the usefulness of medicine and those who worked in the medical arena was called into question, which paved the way for the health care reform of today. For example, there were claims that the work of medical practitioners was not based on "evidence" and was therefore unscientific, and thus could potentially cause harm to patients. This discontent coincided with, and perhaps contributed to, different "crises" in the health care arena, including concerns about varied practices among health care professionals, inefficiencies in the health care system that led to escalating costs, increased wait times, and a lack of accountability and transparency (see Bird, Conrad, & Fremont, 2000; Canadian Association of Emergency Physicians Working Group, 2002).

While Chappell and colleagues (2008) locate this discontent in the 1980s and 1990s, Rothman (1991) locates its roots much earlier. For example, he traces new rules that were brought to medicine during the 1960s and 1970s and the reasons for such changes – mainly "an erosion in trust" and "a decline in the deference given to doctors and to their professional judgments" (p. 10). Such changes, he argues, significantly altered the relationship between doctors and patients, and between medicine and society (p. 3). What resulted was a gradual loss of discretion for doctors. "Nonphysicians" now framed the principles that organized the relationships between doctors and patients, including "judicial decisions, bioethical treatises, and legislative resolutions" (p. 4).

These new rules discussed by Rothman (1991) and the discontent discussed by Chappell et al. (2008) produced many structural changes (Rothman, 1991, p. 85) to all sectors of the health care system and its workers, resulting, in part, in the development of a multiplicity of standards, guidelines, and protocols directed at clinical practice. This production of texts reflected the desire to ensure the efficient and effective management of health care systems and their workers as well as instil notions of accountability in health care practices (Mykhalovskiy & Weir, 2004; Rankin & Campbell, 2006); an era of accountability, coordination, and control emerged, based on the "best" available evidence. Inseparable from this discussion on health reform and restructuring practices in Canada and abroad are ideologies of neoliberalism and new public management, as discussed in chapter 1.

We saw in chapters 2 and 4 the activation of protocols by Julie and Jake when, for example, Julie took out her orange book and quickly referred to it. We also saw the activation of protocols in chapter 3 when Dan and Hanna decided to place their patient on the C-Spine board and when they explained to the nurse their decision to do so. This orange book, representing a new standardized set of protocols, was introduced in Calgary and throughout the province about two weeks before I began my ride-alongs. Known officially as Medical Control Protocols, the protocols are what Timmermans and Berg (2003) call procedural standards. Procedural standards outline which medical interventions paramedics are supposed to do, based on the "presentation" of the patient. According to AHS, these textual technologies provide paramedics with "clearly defined clinical treatment pathways that EMS paramedical staff will follow when providing care. MCPs are NOT guidelines. They are protocols and must be followed."[1] The goal of these protocols, as Rankin and Campbell (2006) explain, is to tidy up "what can otherwise be very divergent treatment practices" and, in doing so, improve the quality of care patients receive and track that improvement (pp. 66–7).

Embedded within these protocols are principles of evidence-based medicine (EBM). According to Mykhalovskiy and Weir (2004), EBM is central to contemporary health care reforms that claim to offer clinicians better tools to support clinical decision making (see also Daly, 2005). EBM instils a scientific rationality in both policy and practice (Hall, 2005) and is central to the justification and accountability of medical practitioners' practices and decision-making (Hunter, 1996, p. 800). The use of protocols in pre-hospital emergency settings, while intended to increase quality of care and improve patient outcomes, also connects to the efficient use of hospital and pre-hospital resources. Rankin and Campbell (2006) explain that the "use of a clinical pathway advances hospital efficiency by standardizing and streamlining the treatment regimens for patients with certain diagnoses" (p. 66). Timmermans and Berg (2003) describe similar intents of protocols, in that they are geared towards providing efficiency, accountability, transparency, and effectiveness to health practice, while also providing "a means of managerial influence over work that previously was regulated professionally" (Rankin & Campbell, 2006, p. 70). Such a shift, according to Dopson and Fitzgerald (2005), can be viewed "as an important lever to ensure clinical practice is more effective and represents value for money" (p. 1).

In this light, while all paramedics are trained based on standards set by the Alberta College of Paramedics (or a similar College elsewhere) and the Paramedic Association of Canada, the protocols are geared towards organizing their work by shaping and restricting what they can and cannot do to their patient and therefore taming their professional discretion. A field trainer and paramedic with over 30 years of experience explained these changes as they entered into her work:

> [In the past] there didn't seem to be any ... standard procedures ... As an EMT you take in your training ... So, then I'm put on an ambulance and I have this sort of book smarts, right, but really not any hands-on experience. So, I'm working with a paramedic that I'm trusting that they know what we need to do, and you learn kind of as you go, but then they all didn't seem to have any real guidelines; it's what they'd been taught in school ... To see that evolve where we seem to have, you know, more of a handle from a medical director's point of view and then actual standard operating procedures or protocols so that people kind of knew we were all on the same page on how to handle any given situation.

One of the primary jobs of medical directors is to develop the protocols. In addition to "overseeing educational programs" and being responsible for "discipline and remedial training," one medical director I spoke with explained how his work connects to EMS protocols:

> So, within the protocols, which is the biggest piece of what we do, it would include selection of drugs, various clinical interventions, standard of practice, scope of practice; all those types of things ... So, really what paramedics do in the field is an extension of emergency medicine or the emergency department out into the field. So, most of their protocols mirror what we do in the emergency department based on current practice, current literature, current evidence.[2]

As alluded to in earlier chapters, while paramedics spoke about the importance of being compliant and not working outside of protocols and their scope of practice, there is much variance in how these procedural standards are accomplished, especially in light of the different types of chief complaints paramedics treat. The protocols were developed with this complexity in mind because, as another director explained, "there are some areas that paramedics address on a daily basis that are not adequately addressed through a single protocol." This complexity was reflected in the "Standard Approach and Ongoing Assessment" protocol that is embedded within each protocol, reflecting that the protocols are designed to "be used either sequentially, independently, or concurrently ... So that's where a little bit of the art comes in ..." We saw the art of medicine reflected in the talk of Jake and Julie in chapter 4 when they described flexing, bending, or using protocols concurrently to meet the needs of their patients. Adding to this complexity, and moving beyond the biomedical artfulness of paramedics' work, we saw throughout chapters 2–4 how paramedics dually, and in continuous ways, orient to the medical and the non-medical contexts of their work, like the social or physical environments. We also see additional complexity in how paramedics do interpretive work with the information from different technologies (e.g., the CAD and medical devices) in ways that skilfully inform their socio-medical gaze and interactions with their patients.

Lastly, the medical directors both explained how protocols are made more multifaceted by having different "drivers" or pathways based on "time spent with the patient." This complexity is evident in attempts to reflect differences in transport times between rural and urban paramedic contexts, while still holding on to the desire to reduce the variability in paramedics' work and the discursive assumption that "human physiology doesn't change, whether you're in an urban centre or a rural centre." As a result, the standardized protocols have "different branches in them based on transport time."

The protocols in Calgary, both the new ones and the old ones, limited what paramedics could do – they could not work to their full scope as determined by the Alberta College of Paramedics. However, with the introduction of the new protocols that are part of current reform processes, the paramedics in this study generally agreed that the protocols allowed them to work closer to their full scope, that is, provide more pre-hospital interventions in terms of treatment, medication, and the use of technology. Julie, for example, described the new protocols as being "more aggressive in our treatments of certain situations ... they're going to force us to think more, they're going to force us to problem solve more, and they're going to force us to have more foresight than what the old protocols did." As the field trainer explained, with the introduction of the new protocols, paramedics in Calgary "gained probably a lot more skill on medications and stuff than we would have normally in the past ... [including] a whole bunch of equipment that was new to us."

While both EMT-Ps and EMTs in Calgary could do more under the newly introduced protocols, the scope of work especially expanded for EMTs, as illustrated during one ride-along where an EMT-P, who also acts as a supervisor, said, "Thank god for the [new] protocol[s]." He explained that with the new protocols, EMTs are now able do more, whereas under the old Calgary protocols, "basically EMTs were not allowed to do anything." Under the old protocols, EMT-Ps did much more of the work than EMTs: "Basically it put 90 per cent of the workload on paramedics [EMT-Ps], just because they refused to allow the EMTs to work to their scope. So that has changed. So now ... as long as it's in her scope of practice [referring to his partner, who is an EMT], she's allowed to take the patient and be responsible for her ..." In doing so, the new protocols shifted some of the work that EMT-Ps do on to EMTs.

One EMT explained how this expanded scope has changed his work in Calgary by giving an example of a patient who was given an IV and saline solution by a paramedic: in the past, "the EMT couldn't be in the back" of the ambulance without the supervision of the EMT-P, whereas now he is "allowed to stay in the back with the patient. But um, a few years ago, a paramedic wouldn't be in the back, no question, just 'cause the drugs were out of the EMT scope." The paramedic supervisor's comment, "Thank god," implied that he was happy to have some of the workload taken off his shoulders. The EMTs I spoke with also seemed to generally like having more responsibility in Calgary.

What I want to emphasize here is that the protocols "hook" paramedics into reform practices geared towards addressing the aforementioned health care crises; they attempt to control and better manage costs by doing more with less while also making their work visibly accountable. This "hook" is facilitated by the introduction of the electronic Patient Care Record (ePCR), which is the focus of the next section. This technology is aimed at not only increasing compliance through its monitoring potential, but also collecting data elements central to making work visible and reforming work based on the knowledge that the technology produces.

The Electronic Patient Care Record (ePCR)

I introduced readers to the ePCR in chapter 2 as an institutional technology that collects standardized information for different individuals or parties of interest based on the interaction between the paramedic practitioner and patient. As such, the ePCR, like all reports, "has a frame that holds it together" (Pence, 2001, p. 211). For example, the technology consists of different screens and dropdown menus that paramedics touch to activate and type and/or tap the information into the device. It is a device that is generally "on their person" throughout the duration of a call. A manager of the ePCR explained that it is an electronic reporting system that captures key information, including the patient's demographic and clinical information. Furthermore, different legislation in the province, such as the Freedom of Information and Protection of Privacy Act, the Health Information Act, and the Emergency Health Services Act, organizes the content collected in it and how the content can be used.

The original ePCR device used by Calgary was developed by ZOLL. According to its website,[3] ZOLL is a "leading provider of solutions that help fire and EMS organizations of all sizes optimize their people, processes, and technology, leading to clinical excellence and business success." In addition to its data-mining ability and "data management solutions," the ePCR, as claimed by ZOLL, collects information from calls that can be managed in order to maximize "business performance." As the ePCR manager in Calgary explained when it was originally introduced, "We expect this new ePCR solution to improve patient care, operational efficiencies and capabilities, as well as improve documentation compliance."[4]

Since AHS took over EMS in 2009, a new ePCR was introduced that is now being used throughout the province in addition to other locales in Canada, the United States, the United Kingdom, the Netherlands, Australia, Brazil, Spain, and Saudi Arabia.[5] The new device is called "Siren ePCR Suite" and is produced by Medusa Medical Technologies. According to its website, and similar to ZOLL, the ePCR is a technology that intends to improve the "speed and accuracy" of recording patient information by providing paramedics "with more efficient data capture tools." The intended goal is to allow "paramedics to spend less time documenting patients' ailments – and more time treating them." Medusa also claims that this ePCR provides a "solution" that "make[s] every second count," facilitates "better patient outcomes," and produces "powerful reports … [to] observe trends, and view statistics to improve agency performance and patient care." The stated potentiality of this technology is to "analyze and effect change." In doing so, according to the website, "evidence-based medicine has never been easier."

While paramedics work closely with the ePCR for "continuity of care" purposes, they also work closely with it, as one paramedic said, "to cover [their] own ass" and because "it can save you" from getting into trouble, since it is a "legal document." Another paramedic whom I spoke with during the pilot study leading up to this research explained that people are cognizant of the "quality control aspect of the PCR … [because] more than anything else it's used to hang them out to dry, to get them into trouble, right" (Corman & Melon, 2014, p. 160). A central managerial theme with the introduction of the ePCR is that, in addition to solving the "problem with documentation" practices (illegibility and incomplete PCRs), it is also aimed at ensuring protocol compliance and producing data of that compliance for quality assurance and performance management and improvement purposes. According to a manager of the ePCR, one of the main reasons why Calgary (and now the province) switched from paper PCRs to electronic PCRs is because "everybody charts a little bit differently … How do you QA [quality assurance] that? … So now you're collecting a standardized set of data, right." As such, the ePCR facilitates data collection and usage, as explained by one medical director, which allows for the monitoring of front-line work more easily than ever before.

[The ePCR] makes it much easier to search for some of these problems. You know back in the day when we had paper charts we would have to manually go through all of these, so it's just a way of streamlining the audit process and actually select the cohort or charts that we're going to review for that specific audit ... From a data management standpoint, [the] ePCR is very useful.

Embedded within the ePCR is a discourse of quality control, which is "central to the managerialist agenda" (Clarke & Newman, 1997, p. 119). Furthermore, central to quality control is quality assurance; in the context of paramedics, this principle is geared towards ensuring that paramedics use evidence-based practices as outlined in the protocols, which are what count as appropriate interventions within their scope of practice. Lastly, these concepts are linked together in an overarching theme of health care reform and restructuring practices of continuous quality improvement, which aim to intervene in "how work is carried out" through "ongoing efforts to measure and improve work processes" (Mykhalovskiy et al., 2008, p. 199). Writing about a different context, Jackson and Slade (2008) link quality assurance to continuous quality improvement, which they define as "a highly technical practice involving the systematic use of an ongoing cycle of planning, executing, checking, and refining operations to improve efficiencies and to eliminate waste in all aspects of the production process" (p. 30). Exemplifying this, the "ePCR Training" document provided to me by a field trainer and used to train paramedics explains that completed ePCRs go to "management (for trending, audits, research), lawyers/court (for legal proceedings, Fatality Inquiries), and Alberta Health and Wellness for monitoring" in order to affect quality change in a continuous manner, and to ensure compliance. The document also explains that documentation is important because "we must comply with EMS national standards as set out by Accreditation Canada." Documents like this reflect the new managerialist agenda in EMS geared towards targeting the work of front-line workers to effect change.

I am interested in how compliance is achieved and the work that goes into producing institutional representations of compliance because these socially organized processes are central to accomplishing the managerial agenda. In the next section, I focus on the work of people and the technologies that interface with their work, which are integral to activating and accomplishing the managerial agenda. Compliance is especially important based on past and present problems of data collection and reporting practices that have been endemic in emergency medical services, as argued in the Review, and current attempts to solve these problems.

Producing Compliance and Quality on the Front Lines

While the ePCR facilitates the use of data to "analyze and effect change," it is the work of people behind the scenes that, in addition to the work of front-line workers, accomplishes this reality, ensuring both compliance with the protocols and the recording of data that demonstrates compliance. These objectives are mainly accomplished through the monitoring or "audit" work of people behind the scenes, as facilitated by and through the ePCR. Field trainers, paramedic supervisors, and medical directors all play a key role in this endeavour.

The work of field trainers is to facilitate the training of paramedics both on and off the streets. Central to this training is monitoring and evaluating compliance of paramedics with their professional standards and protocols. The field trainers I spoke with explained that there are two standardized forms that are used to evaluate the paramedic: the "Field Observation Record" and the "Emergency Medical Services Clinical Case Review." The Field Observation Record, for example, is used by field trainers to see if paramedics are "following the protocols ..." To do this, field trainers will "show up on a call ... [and] follow them to the hospital" and observe what the paramedics "were normally going to do" on the call. After the call is finished, the field trainer will go over the Field Observation Record with the crew.

While field trainers are observing paramedics on an actual call, they orient to the Field Observation Record, which focuses on "a variety of aspects of the call" that are relevant to quality assurance, including safety, assessment, diagnostic testing, and pharmacology skills, clinical decision making, and communication/professionalism. The Record is accompanied by a system where paramedics are scored "on a one to five" point scale based on specific "criteria," where "three is doing what's expected." The field trainer contrasted an "average" score of three with a score of two, which is assigned when a paramedic "missed something that another practitioner of equal scope would have done," and a score of one, where the practitioner "missed multiple areas, and that wasn't good." Scores of one, two, and three were further contrasted with a score of four, where the practitioner "thought outside the box, you've come up with something unique that's outstanding." This field trainer went on to explain that a "four would be that you had done everything as expected for a three, and then ... you know, safety, or skills, or pharmacology, etc, that would give you an example of what might mandate a four. So, it would be going over and above what would be expected." If working above average occurred frequently, a score of five would be assigned.

The Field Observation, which one paramedic supervisor explained is ideally done twice a year for each paramedic, counts a paramedic's work based on standardized institutional expectations. The goal, as the field trainer explained, is to provide paramedics with feedback for learning and development. Unlike the Clinical Case Review (discussed below), "We don't actually even tally up the overall score" of the Field Observation, because this process is primarily used for educational purposes. While the focus is educational, the field trainer also explained that one of the goals is to "see that they're following the protocols." Furthermore, one paramedic explained that this assessment can be used by a supervisor for a paramedic's annual performance review.

The Clinical Case Review examines "a lot of the same things" as the Field Observation, and is based on a similar scoring sheet as described above. However, in contrast to the Field Observation, the Clinical Case Review is typically done four times a year "as a standard" (paramedic supervisor) and "is tallied" with the intent of providing a clinical "snapshot" in order to assess the quality of work of paramedics. Tallying is done by people, usually field trainers, "sitting in an office using the [printed ePCR] document" (field trainer). Essentially, what the field trainer looks for is to see if specific protocols were followed, based on the chief complaint identified. The field trainer exemplified this work when he gave a hypothetical example of a paramedic who, based on his reading of the paramedic's printed ePCR, "gave oxygen to the patient who was short of breath, but it took you 25 minutes to give oxygen." Because the paramedic "held off" on giving the patient oxygen in a "timely" manner, this reflected a "competency" problem due to "bad clinical decision making."

In addition to trying to ensure quality through compliance with protocols, discourses of risk and safety are central to the Clinical Case Review and thus are embedded within the text, which is one of the reasons why ensuring protocol compliance is so important. This became clear when the field trainer gave the example of a court proceeding and a paramedic explaining to the court what she did to a patient that reflected a score of a three on the Case Review as "follow[ing] your

MCPs [protocols]," and therefore as not representing a competency "problem."

Both of these text-mediated events – the Field Observation and the Clinical Case Review – are directed towards instilling compliance and producing knowledge of that compliance that institutionally reflects quality of care. Furthermore, "quality" of care is determined and reflected specifically in the Clinical Case Review as determined by the categories provided in the ePCR and the standardized evaluative document. This logic was expressed by one paramedic supervisor, who might use both the Clinical Case Review and the Field Observation Record as part of the annual performance review of paramedics.

In addition to using these more official documents in assessing the quality of care provided by paramedics to patients, one supervisor explained that, "on occasion," she will review the ePCRs of paramedics, which she can access on her office computer. This supervisor explained, "I'll just look at, you know, thoroughness of the PCR itself, and also I'll look at, you know, what are they documenting …" She explained that she usually does this for "the younger people." Based on these more informal reviews – "I'm not going through it with any formalized process like the CCR [Clinical Case Review]" – she might "put a bug in a field trainer's ear" to alert them that a paramedic might need additional support, which may activate reviews of the paramedic. In both formal and informal methods of reviewing the work of paramedics, this supervisor assumes that she can infer good paramedic practices from good documentation. She made this assumption clear when she said, "To me … documentation does to a certain degree reflect patient care, more ability to provide patient care, and if your documentation sucks, your treatment, I'm a firm believer that your treatment usually sucks." With that said, when the supervisor qualifies her statement by saying, "to a certain degree," it appears that she recognizes that there are divergences between paramedics' actual embodied work on the streets and how it is recorded in the categories embedded within different technological devices.

In addition to field trainers and paramedic supervisors, medical directors are also at work behind the scenes producing compliance. Medical directors, for instance, not only organize what paramedics can and cannot do but also ensure that paramedics' scope of practice is followed. As such, the work of medical directors also connects to quality control and quality assurance practices – safeguarding that what paramedics do is compliant with the legislation, professional bodies that govern their work, and the protocols. This compliance work was made visible when medical directors talked about their role of providing medical oversight.

One medical director described how medical oversight can be divided into three categories, "retrospective, online, and prospective," with retrospective oversight being achieved primarily through the review of ePCRs. Another medical director explained that, in order to do his work of overseeing what paramedics do on the streets, he does "quality assurance audits of specific clinical areas from their patient care records," like "pulling" ePCR records "randomly" and examining them to ensure that what was indicated on the ePCR "was consistent with the protocol that we've designed around that agent." In addition to doing "more broad audits of clinical care," the medical director typically reviews ePCRs that involve "higher acuity," like trauma calls and/or calls when issues come up that "trigger" an audit, such as "time delays" in transferring patients to hospital and complaints from physicians. In addition, he may also review the Clinical Case Reviews completed by field trainers. He does this "when a problem has been identified."

For the higher acuity audits, the medical director explained that he looks for "several key things," like whether the paramedic obtained "demographic information" (name, date of birth, health care number). This information is "the only way we can track [patients]." He also looks to see if the practitioner obtained "a set of vital signs" and whether the vitals were repeated every 10–15 minutes. The goal here is to "see trends" in the patient. Additional information examined includes whether a medical history, chief complaint, and medications were recorded. He looks at the "physical exam" section: "Did they, you know, document the status of the veins on the neck, the position of the trachea, did they listen to the chest, did they palpate the abdomen, so is there a physical exam?"

The final section the medical director looks at is the treatment section. It is this section that makes visible the "protocols or standing orders" and any compliance issues with them. If paramedics are not compliant, he explained, "We try and delve into why they're using [the protocol] inappropriately ... We're trying to identify whether or not this is an individual's or a one-off problem versus a systemic problem which needs a systemic solution." He explained that non-compliance is usually a "training issue"; however, there are times when paramedics "intentionally" do not use the protocols appropriately and therefore "it can become a discipline issue as well."

Closely connected to evaluating the quality of paramedics' work is evaluating the timeliness of their work. While the field trainers might focus on the timeliness of interventions, the amount of time paramedics spend at the scene with the patient, known as "scene time," is also important. As one medical director explained, "A lot of what we do actually involves time-dependent emergencies." With the introduction of the ePCR, time can be monitored more closely than ever before as this technology interfaces with the Computer Aided Dispatch (CAD) technology described in the previous chapter (this will be discussed further in the next section). Time is also a key evaluative feature of the monitoring of paramedics vis-à-vis chief complaint(s) and the protocols. For example, for "time sensitive conditions, like say an acute traumatic injury, a stroke, or a heart attack ... we look for a scene time of 10 minutes or less. For general medical conditions we say 20 minutes or less would be a general target." To assess scene time, the medical director will look at "how much intervention was required" and the context of the call, for example if the patient had to be transported from a "third-story apartment with no elevator." This is where the comments section in the ePCR might come into play, though that field is not mandatory for paramedics to complete.

The comments section is one of the only ways to account for the complexity of what paramedics do outside of the aforementioned categories. According to the provincial ePCR training document, what is "not written ... did not happen!" Even though the comments section favours discourses of biomedicine and accountability similar to what is embedded within the other sections of ePCR, it is less black and white. The complexity that can be made visible in the comments section is oriented to by people at work behind the scenes in determining compliance and quality of care. In other words, while the technologies discussed above are central to the accountability of what paramedics do, and produce very specific knowledge of that work, people who activate these technologies also take into consideration other information, primarily the comments section of the ePCR. When, for example, medical directors look at the context of the call, they "look at what the dialogue is that paramedics have written in with respect to their rationale." Referring to the comments section of the ePCR, "we would look for anything unusual in the patient presentation that would explain why they deviated from protocol or why things were done in a specific order ..."

The work of these individuals behind the scenes is concerned with adherence to the protocols and the biomedical knowledge that is primarily captured in the technologies discussed above. Central to the discourses embedded within the ePCR, including the comments section, and further brought to the fore in the Field Observation Report and the Clinical Case Review, is biomedical and accounting knowledge thought to reflect clinical practice specifically and, more broadly, the work of paramedics. While this knowledge is important, it is in contrast to what counts for paramedics; whereas paramedics spoke of the medical interventions as important, one paramedic described the medical interventions as the "monkey skills" of EMS work. As they oriented to the biomedical knowledge embedded within the protocols, they also oriented beyond the "physiology" and "time" to the actual patient and the unstandardized contexts in which their work occurred.

While the workers behind the scenes qualify the quantitative information garnered from the ePCR and the standardized assessment tools discussed above by reading the comments section, it is the numbers that take precedence in the socially organized production of compliance. This is exemplified in the next section, where we will see that this complexity is obliterated by technologies activated by people that interface with the work practices of paramedics and determine what knowledge gets counted and can be counted, and thus is reportable up the lines of the institutional order.

Business Intelligence – "Analyse and Effect Change"

The information collected in the ePCR and Dispatch Centre is not simply used for monitoring the work of paramedics; it can also be used, according to Medusa, to report on the performance of the EMS system, with the goal of providing "significant clinical and operational benefits to improve performance and quality."[6] The ePCR manager, quality assurance specialist, and performance management specialist are a group of individuals whose job it is to report local actions of paramedics to governing bodies, primarily Alberta Health (AH) and AHS, for continuous quality improvement purposes that inform policy and practice.

The ePCR manager is responsible for overseeing the ePCR system in the province and ensuring that it is compliant with "applicable AHS policy." She explained that there is a team of "integrated technologies people" who "do our quality assurance," ensuring that "pretty specific" information is reported to AH. This information includes the call type, which paramedics were on the call, the "timings of the events," whether or not the patient was transported to the hospital (and if so, which one), and the "treatments and assessments," including medications given, "signs and symptoms, primary impression, [and] chief complaints."

The data from the ePCR is submitted to Alberta Ambulance Information Management System, known as AAIMS, and is based on the "mandatory fields" embedded within the ePCR and time stamps collected from the Dispatch Centre. The required fields are legislated by government (AH, 2012) and involve categories that pertain to "clinical, legal, or financial requirement ... So, things like response outcome, times, call types, signs and symptoms, primary impression [of the patient], all that stuff [is] mandatory" (ePCR manager) (see figure 7.1 for a summary of some of the information collected and reported to government).

The performance management specialist described his work of data management and reporting as primarily tracking the work of paramedics "on a day-to-day," "month-to-month," and "quarterly basis."[7] Information reported on includes both operational information and clinical information. The operational "pillar" of information includes reports that pertain to "the delivery of resources to the frontlines ... basically what EMS is doing in terms of everything from volume to our response times and that goes all the way up to the Ministry of Health." He explained that his work of reporting is geared towards not simply monitoring front-line workers but also making their work visible "in a consumable" or reportable "format" based on data from both the CAD and ePCR. The "daily reports," for example, are sent to paramedic supervisors about their staff, and include things like "call volume they're generating, their performance around response times, the time that they're spending at hospitals, all that kind of thing."

In addition, and in order to identify trends that can be used for operational purposes, the statistics are broken down, according to the performance management specialist, into "lights and sirens and non-emerge" calls at "the 50th percentile ... [the] median of your response data" and the "90th percentile," which refers to the response time of ambulance units that occurs 90 per cent of the time or less. It was explained to me that the 90th percentile "is a good indication of where some of your long responses are and your overall distribution," which is "really important data to operations" because trends can be identified. From this information, "operational decisions" can be made; the intent of these "true performance measures" is to understand "where our resources are getting tied up and therefore where we have to ... Deployment has to shift accordingly to that, so ..."

7.1 AAIMS data collected

Core Date Elements:

- PCR number
- Date of Service
- License Number
- No Transport
- No Transport Reason

Other information collected includes:

- **Incident Information** – This section contains the core and main information of the PCR.
- **Attendant Information** – This section contains the information on Attendants A, B, and C.
- **Patient Information** – This section contains the personal information about the patient.
- **Times Information** – This section contains the response times for the PCR event.
- **Vital Signs** – This section contains the results of each time the vitals are taken.
- **Skilled Intervention** – This section describes the treatment and medication given and by which attendant.
- **Observation Information** – This section contains any additional information not listed in the incident or response information.
- **Trip Information** – This section contains information about response and transport types and latitude and longitude of the trip.

(AH, 2012, pp. 7, 19)

Whereas the operational component of data collection and reporting results in commensurable information that is interpreted institutionally as "what the fleet is doing, how long they're with patients," the other data reported – the second "pillar" of data collection and reporting – primarily comes from the ePCR and represents the "clinical portion" of performance management. The specialist explained that, since the introduction of the ePCR, the clinical information has played an increasingly important role compared with the operational data because "obviously the amount of data that's going along with that is significant … There's appetites for both of the data, but we're starting to, I would say arguably we're really getting exposed to, the clinical side more and more."

The specialist went on to explain that the electronic form of the data created by the ePCR has made it possible to readily use the data in ways that were not possible in the past. This electronic data is specifically useful for quality assurance purposes; "We're starting to build certain methods and certain approaches around developing benchmarks looking at performance measures,"[8] including "activity [operational] measures" and "clinical measures … and a lot of back and forth has been going on with the consultation with the medical directors and the senior executive to figure out what [is] best."

While the potentiality of data collection and processing is strengthened by reform practices, there are problems with AAIMS and the ePCR as data collection tools, as expressed by both the ePCR manager and the Review of EMS operations (HQCA, 2013). For example, the ePCR manager explained that while "AAIMS was developed to give us reports to tell us how we're doing in our business … AAIMS is not a friend in my book …" This person explained that the database is antiquated and "built on a model we used 15–20 years ago." This sentiment was also expressed by the Review, which claimed that the AAIMS data is "incomplete due to poor data submission compliance and insufficient data quality checks," not to mention "Limited patient care data." As a result, "The provincial EMS data are not currently adequate to be used for comprehensive performance and quality and safety management" (HQCA, 2013, p. 7).

Furthermore, the quality assurance specialist explained that when the categories embedded in the ePCR are not being filled out properly, it makes reporting on EMS happenings challenging. The specialist specifically mentioned the "impression Code" part of the ePCR – a drop-down menu of "probably ten choices" – which she described as the "cause of the call." While the field is "mandatory" to fill out, it is often "overridden" by paramedics. This conflicts with her work because without the field selected she cannot "figure out things, like how many strokes we're going on … what protocol we're using, and how we're treating the patient, and based on what the paramedic was thinking … "

Some people I spoke to discussed the problem of documentation as a "cultural" issue with EMS. However, the specialist, who is also trained as a paramedic with street experience, voiced a disjuncture whereby information required from the ePCR to fulfil data reporting requirements does not match the non-standard work of what paramedics do. Hence, paramedics are selecting non-reportable categories in the ePCR, like "other." This discussion connects to the work of Bakhtin (1986), who differentiates between primary and secondary speech genres, with the former arising from local experiences and the latter being more text-mediated and ideological (Smith, 2005, p. 86): "These primary genres are altered and assume a special character when they enter into complex [secondary] ones. They lose their immediate relation to the actual reality and to the real utterances of others" (Bakhtin, 1986, p. 62). For example, shifting between secondary speech genres of quality assurance language and the primary speech genres reflective of her actual experience of being a paramedic, the specialist explained:

> To audit a protocol is very difficult ... A paramedic rarely is going to go OK, this box, yeah, filled, done, this box, yeah, done. They're going to go OK, well this happened here, and so I might need to go into another protocol and I might need to work with them simultaneously, so it's very hard to audit a specific protocol.

The quantitative data required for auditing purposes is in tension with the complex work of paramedics, and this tension therefore extends beyond being simply a cultural issue. The tension in data collection practices is compounded by the limits of the ePCR, which cannot report on "text fields [including the chief complaint and the comments section] ... we can only audit the drop-down boxes in ePCR ... we can't even pull and report on [those fields]."

Nevertheless, since EMS in Calgary were amalgamated by AHS, there has been a renewed focus on quality assurance and on data collection and processing practices, which connects to the production of compliance discussed above, aimed at producing "robust data management systems" in order to facilitate better management and coordination of EMS (HQCA, 2013, p. 7). It is the work of people behind the scenes, facilitated by different institutional technologies, to try and solve the data collection problems in the province.

In addition to collecting and reporting on the performance of the system, embedded within the ePCR Siren Suite is a "reporting solution" that the performance management specialist described as a "business intelligence tool ... called Cognos" that has the ability to "marry" together different data sources (e.g., human resource data, clinical data, and operational data) and "translate" them.[9] According to IBM, this software produces "reports, analysis, dashboards and scorecards to monitor business performance, analyze trends and measure results ... giv[ing] you the information you need to make better decisions."[10] In addition to analysing data in order to make better decisions that "achieve better business outcomes,"[11] the tool also allows "the business user to analyze facts and anticipate strategic implications by simply shifting from viewing data to performing more advanced predictive or what-if analysis."[12]

Exemplifying the potential of this reporting solution, the importance of having "valid" data, and how knowledge is being used to drive reform practices, the ePCR manager explained that "I want to ... start thinking about incorporating our data into prediction models." This person referred to the Community Health and Pre-hospital Support (CHAPS) program, now implemented in Alberta, as an example.[13] The aim of the CHAPS program is to divert seniors away from hospitals by providing them the "right" service at the "right" time. The ePCR manager explained:

> For example, seniors that are at home, maybe we transport too many seniors to the hospital and they don't need to go to the hospital, right? Maybe what we need to do is increase the medics' scope of practice so that they can treat these people at home more effectively ... maybe if the medic had the ability to prescribe a certain set of medications, he would just call the physician and say: "Here's grandma, she's presenting like this, difficulty urinating, I think she's got a UTI [urinary tract infection], how about if we start her on a seven-day course and see where it takes us?" He'll probably say yes, right?

The study that led to the implementation of this program, as Julie understood it, tried "to prove if we can assess patients in homes ... [The study is] the embryonic form of us doing referrals." "Doing referrals," as Julie mentions, connects to the introduction of protocols that some emergency medical services in North America and elsewhere are considering introducing (or have introduced) in order to alleviate the "inappropriate" use of emergency department resources for patients deemed non-emergent by allowing paramedics to "treat and refer" or "see and treat" their patient rather than transporting them to the hospital (see Finn et al., 2013). Both the ePCR manager and the performance management specialist envisioned future endeavours similar to the CHAPS program where knowledge technologies could be used to "predict" and target areas "where we're having our most [serious] issues" (ePCR manager). In addition to relying on patient-centred logics of providing the "right" service to patients as a justification for such reforms, the ePCR manager also relied on business and accounting logics when he explained that "every" health care system, "Alberta's not immune," is doing this to save money – "It's all about trying to reduce how much money it takes to treat people …"

Tracing Relations of Governance and Accountability

I now map some of the key knowledge processes central to the work of paramedics and other workers in the EMS system as a whole. The purpose of mapping how things work is to show how knowledge is socially organized through institutional and social processes. According to Smith (2005), "A map assembles different work knowledges, positioned differently, and should include, where relevant, an account of the texts coordinating work processes in institutional settings" (p. 226). My goal here is to make more explicit how individuals orient to similar or different knowledge processes depicted in this and previous chapters (figures 7.2 and 7.3). I also aim to depict how knowledge-production processes in EMS gear up the institutional ladder of accountability and governance (figure 7.4).

Figures 7.2 and 7.3, which are interrelated, depict knowledge processes at work that individuals orient to. These knowledge processes seek to address two interconnected questions: 1) What resources are needed to address the current emergency? and 2) Is the system being managed efficiently and effectively in real time and based on records of past activities? Figure 7.2 answers question 1 by exemplifying how individuals orient to real-time knowledge geared towards dealing with an actual emergency. This knowledge process collects and distributes information about the emergency to different front-line workers. We see in this diagram that different workers orient to real-time information in complementary yet different ways.

Figure 7.3 answers question 2 by depicting how individuals in EMS orient to knowledge processes that are geared towards managing EMS efficiently and effectively vis-à-vis real-time decision making (RTDM) and records of past activities (ROPAs) by providing valid data to assess performance at the individual and system level. Corollary to assessing the performance is the "effective" management and oversight of the system and its workers, which also requires specific data. We see in this knowledge process that similar data can have different managerial readings, depending on the task/orientation of the one reading the text. Also, data collected from the real-time knowledge process discussed above are sometimes read and used for supervisory purposes. Other information is produced specifically for managerial purposes, like providing generalized/aggregated understandings of what is going on in the city for the purposes of allocating resources. In addition, information about the paramedic might be produced for supervisory purposes (e.g., discipline, annual performance review, education, and training).

Figures 7.2 and 7.3 represent how the work and knowledge processes described in the previous chapters "blend" into the work and knowledge production practices described in this chapter. It is at the Dispatch Centre, for example, where much of the tracking of time for paramedics occurs (the ePCR can also "time-stamp" interventions by paramedics). Furthermore, the work of individuals discussed in this chapter aims, in part, to manage the work of paramedics and facilitate the production of text-mediated representations of compliance and quality through different knowledge technologies they have available to them, such as the ePCR, Field Observation Record, Clinical Case Reviews, and data reports.

The goal of how knowledge is being put together is to monitor and account for the work of paramedics while also ensuring and making visible the quality of EMS. We see in this chapter that information collected for some purposes is also used for other purposes, like producing performance measures of time, indicators of quality assurance, and business intelligence endeavours. As such, knowledge produced in some places is "carried on primarily in a textual mode" to other institutional sites (Smith, 2005, p. 178). Figure 7.4 (discussed below) represents how some of the information produced from different knowledge technologies is further passed along to governing bodies such as AH and AHS for the purposes of monitoring, reforming, and restructuring. In addition to AH and AHS relying on this information for governance purposes, AHS has enlisted accreditation bodies, like Accreditation Canada, to assist in its project of governance and to help instil a "culture" of continuous quality improvement.[14]

According to Accreditation Canada, accreditation is a process whereby accreditors inspect "some aspects of a client's operations"

7.2 Orienting to the here and the now of an emergency

Dispatch Centre
• Real-time information passed on to paramedics, hospital staff and managers
• Is this the right chief complaint?
• Is the scene safe?
• REPAC

Paramedics
• Continuity of care
• Treating the patient not the protocol
• What equipment do I need?
• Where am I going?
• Is the scene safe?
• Type, quality, and notes of call?
• "REPAC please"

Paramedic Supervisor
• Alert Status in Calgary?

ED Physician
• What was done to the patient and why?
• Other "comments" from the paramedic

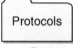

Protocols

ePCR and CAD

Triage Nurse
• What brought the patient in today?
• Relevant clinical information
• Do I trust the paramedic?
• Can the patient be put into the waiting room?
• What type of bed should I assign the patient?
• How are we on hospital resources (e.g. beds)?

Unit Nurse
• Can I have a more detailed description of what happened?
• Relevant clinical information

Patient
• What is wrong with me?
• Do I really need to go to the hospital?
• Which hospital are we going to?

with the goal of informing "health care leaders, organizations, and governments on key health care issues arising from accreditation."[15] This is accomplished through Accreditation Canada's "Qmentum" program, which offers "powerful tools" of measurement – "The importance of measurement cannot be understated in quality improvement ..." (Accreditation Canada, 2011, p. 16) – such as "required organizational practices" or ROPs, which include "evidence-based,"[16] onsite surveys by accreditation personnel and organizational self-surveys, to evaluate the performance of health care systems/organizations.

7.3 Management of EMS in real time and through records of past activities

Field Trainer
• Is the paramedic compliant? [ROPAs]
• Where is paramedic struggling? [ROPAs]
• How can we improve paramedic's performance? [ROPAs]

Triage Nurse
• CTAS score? [ROPAs and RTDM]

AHS
• "Solve problem of documentation" [ROPAs]
• QI and QA [ROPAs]

Courts
• Legal Proceedings [ROPAs]
• "Dd you follow your MCPs?" {ROPAs}

Medical Director
• Are paramedics compliant? [ROPAs]
• QA and higher acuity "audits" (e.g. was the work timely?) [ROPAs]
• What happened? [ROPAs]
• Who is at fault (individual or system)? [ROPAs]
• Timeliness [ROPAs]
• Online Medical Consulation [RTDM]

Paramedic Supervisor
• How did the paramedic perform annually? [ROPAs]
• Are paramedics compliant? [ROPAs]
• Do paramedics have any educational needs? [ROPAs]

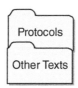

Protocols

Other Texts

ePCR and CAD

Quality Assurance Specialist
• What are the paramedics doing? [ROPAs]
• Is data being collected "valid"? {ROPAs}

Paramedics
• Billing [ROPAs]
• "It can save you" – Quality Assurance [ROPAs]

Dispatch Centre
• How do the resources in the City look? [RTDM]
• Do I need to flex? [RTDM]
• Time is of the essence [ROPAs and RTDM]

Performance Management Specialist
• What is the fleet doing? [RTDM and ROPAs]
• What are paramedics doing? [ROPAs]
• Reports on a daily, monthly, and quarterly basis? [ROPAs]
• How can we use data to predict services and target "issue" areas? [ROPAs]
• Timeliness [ROPAs]

ePCR Specialist
• Is information collected compliant with AHS policy? [ROPAs]
• How can we use data to predict services and target "issue" areas? {ROPAs}

◊ **ROPAs** – record of past activities
◊ **RTDM** – real-time decision making

7.4 Reporting performance

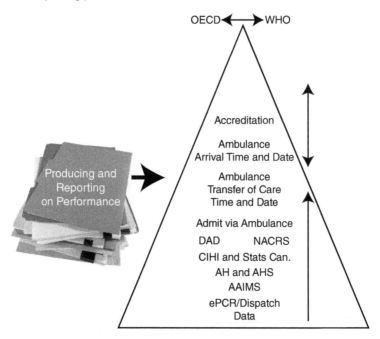

The process of accreditation emphasizes discourses of "health system performance, risk prevention planning, client safety, performance measurement, and governance," all of which are geared towards increasing the accountability and quality of health care systems[17] in order to produce "'high-performing' organizations" (Accreditation Canada, 2011, p. 10). As such, a key focus of accreditation is on ensuring patient safety and ensuring that the "philosophy of continuously improving the quality of care and services is also incorporated" in health care systems.[18] Essential to accreditation processes is the underlying assumption that performance measures "help organizations in their [continuous] quality improvement efforts" (Accreditation Canada, 2009, p. 10). Furthermore, by having a standard set of performance measures throughout Canada (and elsewhere), Accreditation Canada can monitor "health care performance measures used at the federal, provincial, and territorial levels" (p. 10).

Connected to the focus on accreditation are different national and international health services research organizations, specifically the

Canadian Institute of Health Information (CIHI), the Organisation for Economic Cooperation and Development (OECD), and the World Health Organization (WHO). According to Rankin and Campbell (2006), "health services research is a highly applied multidisciplinary field of research that addresses the structure, process, delivery and organization of health services (Mykhalovskiy 2001). It relies on quantitative and positivist research methods using complex statistical analysis to establish relationships between health services rendered and health outcomes for a broad selection of populations and services" (p. 192, n. 4). The OECD and WHO in particular "have taken an international lead in encouraging health system performance measurement" geared towards identifying and managing problems in health care and increasing "productivity" of health care systems (Kelley & Hurst, 2006, p. 9, 10).[19]

Figure 7.4 represents how data is funnelled into these organizations. This figure is meant to depict how productions of performance (the left side) in EMS are funnelled up institutional chains of accountability (the right side). The right side of the diagram begins with ePCR/Dispatch Centre data that is submitted to the AAIMS data collection system, as discussed earlier in this chapter. Data collected in AAIMS is submitted to AHS and AH, who then submit particular information to CIHI. The unidirectional black arrow represents how information is passed up this knowledge process to these bodies of governance.

CIHI has two "metadata" databases that capture a multiplicity of information, some of which is specific to EMS. For example, the Discharge Abstract Database (DAD) "captures administrative, clinical and demographic information on hospital discharges (including deaths, sign-outs and transfers)."[20] DAD captures one data element that seems to be unique to pre-hospital emergency health services, "Admit (to hospital) via Ambulance."[21] The National Ambulatory Care Reporting System (NACRS) is the other "metadata" database that "contains data for all hospital-based and community-based ambulatory care."[22] Data elements captured through this database specific to pre-hospital emergency health services include ambulance arrival at hospital time and date, ambulance transfer of care to hospital time and date, and admit via ambulance.[23] Along with Statistics Canada, data elements such as these are submitted to OECD. According to CIHI:

CIHI and Statistics Canada worked together to develop the Canadian segment of the Organisation for Economic Co-operation and Development (OECD) Health Database. Its purpose is to collect and process a consistent series of internationally comparable data for close to 1,200 variables. The OECD Health Database is used to support policy planning, decision-making and research, and facilitates international comparative reporting.[24]

The bidirectional black arrow in figure 7.4 (right side) from AH and AHS to CIHI, Accreditation, OECD, and WHO represents how information is dually funnelled into these bodies of governance and back into processes of reform and continuous quality improvement.

Taken together, these three diagrams depict knowledge processes central to what counts institutionally and for whom. These diagrams also illustrate how what gets counted is constructed from a displaced and subsumed text-mediated caricature of the everyday work of front-line workers and the work of individuals they interface with. In figure 7.2, for instance, we see how different people orient to their work settings, albeit in complementary and sometimes divergent ways in relation to a medical emergency. Technological governance is central to making visible (and invisible) the relevant aspect of work that discursively resonates with institutional ways of knowing, as depicted in figure 7.3. What gets counted in figure 7.3 further connects to figure 7.4 as knowledge is passed up the ladder of institutional accountability and reporting. Processes of governance connected to reform and restructuring practices are central to these diagrams, particularly figures 7.2 and 7.3, whereby "numerically-based forms of expertise" are produced for the purposes of governing "social life" (Mykhalovskiy, 2001, p. 269).[25]

Discussion and Conclusion

In this chapter, I explored how the work of paramedics is being targeted by new forms of managerial control through protocols, the ePCR, quality assurance, and data production processes, all of which are integral to restructuring practices. I discussed how protocols do not act on their own. Rather, they are activated by people at work, including front-line workers, their managers, and other individuals behind the scenes of EMS. Part of the work of the individuals discussed in this chapter is to ensure the compliance of front-line workers in using the protocols appropriately and following appropriate documentary practices in order to produce evidence of that compliance. The ePCR was discussed to exemplify an institutional technology that not only facilitates compliance, through the ability to monitor the work of paramedics more easily than ever before, but also acts as a data collection and processing tool. By focusing on how the work of paramedics is being targeted by technologies of knowledge and governance, my goal was to explicate the social organization of knowledge in EMS by describing how things work.

While I focused on the work of monitoring paramedics, it is important to note that compliance is also achieved through the compelling discourse of EBM and the scientific rationality that is part of the claim that protocols lead to improved quality of care – doing the right thing to the right patient at the right time – while also limiting "risk," both to patients and paramedics. Paramedics buy into this discourse, which was alluded to by many of the paramedics I spoke with and exemplified by Julie and Jake in chapters 2 and 4 in their talk about the importance of not working outside of protocols and in the seriousness in how they write about their work in the ePCRs and the specific audiences they write to, including doctors and lawyers. The language they used, as discussed in earlier chapters, carries social organization; this social organization is made more visible by examining the work of individuals behind the scenes and the accounting and coordinative technologies with which their work interfaces.

As suggested above, the technologies discussed in this and earlier chapters are not only coordinating the work of paramedics but are also producing socially organized knowledge or virtual realities of key performance measures. These measures include efficiency, effectiveness, and accountability of the EMS system based on accounting logics, which are central to reform and restructuring practices. This official reporting of work objectifies and generalizes what paramedics actually do on the streets and opens up their work to continuous quality improvement endeavours based on very specific objectified forms of knowing that are constructed as "evidence" (Rankin & Campbell, 2006, p. 128). What is counted, or the official reporting of what counts, is an ideological or conceptual practice of power (Smith, 1990), a practice that, as Pence (2001) points out, is "circular" (p. 213).

The diagrams in this chapter depict how paramedics and other front-line health care workers "are connected into the extended social relations of ruling and economy and their intersections" (Smith, 2005, p. 29). I focused specifically on information-production practices, data-reporting requirements, and institutional expectations/interests described in this and earlier chapters. These diagrams, therefore, show how texts "anchor" the embodied work of paramedics and other front line-workers in "accountable" ways "within an administrative process"

(Smith, 2005, p. 177). By focusing on key institutional features central to the achievement of what counts as knowledge on the front lines of emergency health services, we see how information collected throughout this socially organized process is put together.

Central to the technologies doing the counting are discourses of business logics aimed at doing more with less. This was exemplified in the predictive potential of the business intelligence tools that are entering into policy and practice. The performance management specialist is essentially hoping to be able to use institutional technologies to identify "where our resources are getting tied up" and, as the ePCR manager explained, target those areas in a predictive, real-time way to create more resources without actually creating more resources. The goal is to limit or divert those who would have in the past gained access to those resources, under the adage of providing the right care to the right patient at the right time. This constitutes a redirection of services for patients that paramedics that I spoke to seemed to agree was a better use of EMS. As such, reducing costs is central to the notion of putting the right patient in the right place at the right time, which was also evident in the Dispatch Centre, where paramedics and patients were directed to the "most appropriate" resource, and technologies were used to allocate the best use of health care resources.

While trying to reduce costs is not problematic in and of itself, what I have made visible here and in the last chapter is some of the work of individuals in EMS, and the different technologies they interface with, in targeting the work of front-line paramedics and creating knowledge of that work. Such knowledge production processes capture only snippets of what actually happens on the front lines of EMS. For example, most of the data captured in the ePCR, reported to AAIMS, and further passed up the institutional chain of accountability to CIHI and OECD are codified data or "core data elements" that only include quantifiable categories. In fact, central to the ideological appearance of "objective" and "valid" data that are reportable and actionable is the quantitative representation described above as produced through the ePCR and technologies at the Dispatch Centre. The work described in this chapter and the technologies central to that work are tied together in terms of quality assurance and continuous quality improvement endeavours geared towards training practitioners, ensuring their safety, ensuring that patients receive quality care, and addressing a main managerial concern in EMS of predicting the unpredictable demand of services in the most efficient and effective ways.

Chapter Eight

Conclusion

What Counts and for Whom?

Throughout parts 1 and 2 of this book, I have explored the work processes of paramedics and other EMS personnel and have begun to explicate how front-line EMS work is organized and coordinated by different institutional technologies in light of changes to how EMS is being organized and restructured. In doing so, I have shed light on how the work of paramedics interfaces with that of other front-line workers, like doctors, nurses, and dispatchers, with their non-standard patients, and with the different technologies central to this interface. I have also illustrated how paramedics' work comes to be known and hooked into different work processes elsewhere in the EMS system and the different institutional technologies central to this "hooking" process. Corollary to this hooking process is the very important question, "How is knowledge in EMS being put together?" These analytical interests have resulted in a close examination of how the work setting of paramedics is socially organized and the knowledge process central to their work setting. Hence, this book is not only about the work of paramedics but also about how managerial technologies are slowly but surely reorganizing that work, often with hidden consequences, and how knowledge of that work is socially structured.

This exploration of knowledge processes raises a very important question: What counts and for whom? In EMS we can see how institutional accounts of work – what becomes institutional knowledge – are put together in a way that displaces and subsumes the actual work of paramedics; the work of paramedics, call-takers, dispatchers, and other workers is "eclips[ed]" (Smith, 1987) or "annihilated actually" (Burns,

1994) by highly specialized and simplified knowledge. For example, the knowledge collected through the Dispatch Centre and the ePCR all becomes a "key organizational element in taking action" and makes up the institutional representation of what counts (Pence, 2001, p. 203). The chief complaint, for instance, and its corresponding protocol determine relevant information collected and made visible. The final reporting of events reflects this discursively organized framing of the event – "the report orients to and is effective in terms of the [chief complaint] ... [The] information is confined to the boundaries set by the schema ..." (pp. 213, 215). This highly organized knowledge process is an abstraction and a textually displaced version of people's doings – "'what is going on' is not as important as 'what happened'" (p. 200).

The rationalities embedded within reform and restructuring practices "directly shape what counts as 'health care' or at the very least what counts as a health-care priority" (Cribb, 2008, p. 237; Clarke & Newman, 1997, p. 66). What is counted then "reflects the concerns of the institution" (Pence, 2001, p. 203). By explicating key processing interchanges, we see how knowledge is produced and also what is missing, in contrast to what is made visible, through this empirical investigation. Information is collected and knowledge is created for specific purposes of governance that subsume and dominate the local interests of paramedics, their patients, and other front-line workers. Through my analysis in part 2, I explicated the knowledge processes central to what institutionally counts, and the technologies central to the demarcation of what is not counted. As a project of discovery, this book has begun to explicate *what is going on* for paramedics on and off the streets in the age of technological governance.

Cause for Concern?

Central to reforms that are targeting EMS in Alberta, and elsewhere, are neoliberal ideologies that seek "value for money" (Rankin & Campbell, 2006, p. 8). The assumption is that, as one person I spoke with said, "We have more demand right now than we have resources to respond to it," and hence there is a need to manage costs rather than create additional resources. As such, technologies of knowledge and governance are being used not only to organize and coordinate the front-line work of paramedics and others but also to create knowledge of that work for purposes of creating efficiencies. As depicted throughout this book, the knowledge that gets constructed and hence "known" as paramedics' work and EMS happenings is an abstracted textual representation based on discursive notions of quality and efficiency. As Mykhalovskiy and colleagues (2008) point out, this text-mediated, "numerically constituted terrain obscure[s] the complexity of health reform as experienced by patients and providers" (p. 198). The problem is that such representations are simplistic; how knowledge is socially organized and put together constructs the work of EMS personnel both on and off the streets as if their work is stepwise and predictable. As my research shows, the work of paramedics is anything but simple and stepwise. Rather, their work is structured by and responsive to a multiplicity of social and political processes that occur within an environment – on the streets – that is, as Jake described it in chapter 5, "predictably unpredictable."

In a similar light, Anselm Strauss and colleagues (1985) suggest that "reform without prior understanding can only lead to ineffectual reform, or even to measures that make matters worse" (p. x). Researchers who have studied front-line health work, for instance, have drawn attention to how reform and restructuring practices leave in their path "hidden dangers" (Rankin & Campbell, 2006); there are consequences for both patients and practitioners that remain invisible to institutional representations of what is being counted or the ideological practices organizing those representations. As my research unfolded, and as is illustrated throughout the previous chapters, I made visible some of the consequences for front-line workers and those they care for that did not show up in the knowledge processes connected to reform and restructuring practices. These consequences are discussed in more detail below.

Doing More with Less

Characteristic of reforms in Alberta is increased pressure on paramedics to do more with less, or at least to do more with the same amount of resources. Technologies like REPAC and the ePCR, the newly introduced protocols, and policies like the waiting room download criteria and flexing are being used to make the system "more efficient." The REPAC technology, for instance, is geared towards directing paramedics to the "most appropriate" hospital, the ePCR is being used to collect data not only for patient care but also in order to provide "business intelligence" to restructure EMS, and the waiting room download criteria are being used to expand resources by downloading patients into the waiting room in order to free up EMS resources.

What are some of the consequences of using coordinative technologies to increase efficiency? We saw in chapter 3 a consequence of reform practices geared towards getting paramedics out of the hospital faster. I gave an example of what I came to understand as paramedics playing a patient up or down and the conflict (e.g., distrust) that can result between paramedics and nurses. We also saw other consequences in the Dispatch Centre; in an attempt to better manoeuvre and utilize resources through REPAC, the trust paramedics develop on the front line with other front-line workers can be eroded, not to mention the additional worries expressed by some patients in being brought to a hospital far away from their place of residence and social support. Such examples illustrate a cost of reforms geared towards neoliberal notions of efficiency whereby some might benefit (e.g., the system) but others might not (e.g., paramedics and patients). In the latter example, cost savings are garnered from the "home sphere" (Rankin & Campbell, 2006, p. 75) by placing more responsibility onto patients and their families to get to the most "appropriate" hospital, even if it is outside their locale of comfort, a burden that is likely to be felt more by those who have the least amount of resources, such as family members who rely on public transit. This cost-saving technique also impacts nurses and paramedics because rapport between them is effaced, which can have direct consequences for patient care, as we saw in chapter 3. These reform and restructuring practices, and the governance technologies that facilitate them, can consequentially shift blame and responsibility onto front-line workers and patients while also creating divisions and tensions among workers, ultimately resulting in making the system more complex and fragmented (Light, 2001).

Connected to this discussion of doing more with less is a concern that some paramedics expressed to me about the increased role that inexperienced paramedics were playing in the city. With that said, some paramedics welcomed the expanded roles of EMTs in the city because it took some of the work off them. Nevertheless, the practice of using less skilled, lower-paid workers (e.g., on-calls and EMTs) is not unique to health care but a "tendency under capitalism" to save costs (Ducey, 2009, p. 96). The expanded scope of practice for EMTs in Calgary is the product of the new provincial protocols that allow less-trained workers to do more. In chapter 5, I briefly discussed how the use of "casuals" can make it difficult to develop rapport between paramedic partners.

As one paramedic who is in a managerial role explained, this can lead to consequences:

> We know that being a paramedic is a stressful job, and we know having confidence in your partner and their skills and abilities in terms of decision making, in terms of clinical procedures, managing a scene, whatever that is, can directly impact how comfortable and confident you feel, and therefore how stressed or unstressed you feel as you go to different scenarios … Casuals have a tough role to fill, because they don't establish that rapport … and that creates sometimes some tension amongst the partnership …

Prior to AHS taking over EMS in Calgary, in order to mitigate the lack of trust and the potentially negative consequences that might result, the city had restrictions so that "no casual [EMT-Ps] could be in charge of an ambulance." In light of reform practices and the discourse "We are one," the same paramedic explained that casuals are being used more in the city, including casual EMT-Ps.

> So, what we're learning now that we're part of health … you're a paramedic, the department has said you passed your interview and you did your protocol training, so you're in charge of the truck, including casuals, and so that's one of the things we're actually, again, interesting to have the interview today. We are right now for the first time in however many years notifying all of our casual paramedics that they will start to be utilized as a stand-alone paramedic on an ambulance with potentially a brand new EMT.

Standards set by the city prior to amalgamation are now being eroded in order to do more with less. This new policy ignores the importance of partner work and of on-the-ground experience that, according to many of the more experienced paramedics I spoke with, set EMS in the city apart from other services.

This deterioration of services also connects to a change in the level of service offered in Calgary that is potentially "coming down the pipes," as one paramedic put it. Many paramedics, for example, spoke to me about how they were concerned that the level of service that made EMS in the city of Calgary, in part, a "Cadillac" service was going to be downgraded. One of their concerns was that EMS in Calgary was going to change from an Advanced Life Support (ALS) service, where all units in the city have, at a minimum, an EMT-P and an EMT, to a Basic Life Support (BLS) service, which requires a minimum of an EMT and an emergency medical responder (EMR) for an ambulance unit. One manager of paramedics expressed this concern when he spoke about how a downgraded system does not reflect the work orientations of paramedics geared towards the potentialities – the "what ifs" – of their work settings and the non-standard patients they meet and treat on the front lines. He said:

> … if I send BLS to everything, but now one of those calls occurs where ALS critical intervention needs to occur, and I've dispatched BLS to it because of what, again, the sender, and the receiver, and that whole 90-second conversation on the phone evaluating what was going on, and we've sent a BLS unit because we've determined it to be X, but now ALS, it turns out that wasn't accurate information because the caller didn't answer the questions correctly or whatever, now I'm another 10 minutes to get ALS on-scene.

While he explained that the majority of calls paramedics go to are categorized as BLS calls, this manager is more concerned with the non-standard potentiality of the work settings of paramedics and the safety of patients than the cost orientation of the service that is being organized solely by a *trust in numbers* (Porter, 1995).

Changing Professional Mandate

Reforms that are geared towards doing more with less connect to restructuring practices in Alberta that target the scope of practice for paramedics in Calgary. With the expanded scope, policies and processes are being put in place that allow paramedics, in some circumstances, to divert patients away from the hospital, and thus avoid "costly" transports. The Community Health and Pre-hospital Support (CHAPS) program, for example, supports expanding the sphere of responsibility for paramedics, a change that is imbued with efficiency logics and encapsulated by the discourse of quality care, at least as it was alluded to by the ePCR manager and performance management specialist (see chapter 7). Connecting to the CHAPS program are future plans for a "treat and refer" policy. For example, according to a policy document by Alberta Health Services (2010b) entitled "Becoming the Best: Alberta's 5-year Health Action Plan, 2010–2015," the government

plans to "expand the role of emergency medical technicians and paramedics to: Treat patients on-site instead of taking them to an emergency
department, as appropriate."[1] In potentially narrowing "what counts"
as an emergency, such reforms are intended to better utilize the current
resources by directing front-line work towards "real" emergencies. In
an "update" on the progress of reforms in the province, Alberta Health
confirms that CHAPS "has been rolled out across the Province" and
that additional protocols have been introduced to allow paramedics to
"treat patients on-scene without transporting them to hospital."[2]

Such restructuring practices are changing the professional mandate
of paramedics. At the time this research was conducted, it was the mandate of paramedics, for the most part, to transport a patient to the hospital whether they were considered a "good" patient or not. Now the
view is that "30 per cent of our call volume doesn't require the hospital"
(medical director), and paramedics are potentially being tasked with
the role of rationing resources. In light of trying to avoid the "wasteful"
use of health care resources, will the work orientations of paramedics geared towards the "what ifs" of providing care to non-standard
patients and work environments be displaced or subsumed by more
"evidence-based" technologies that objectify, generalize, and standardize patients? Jake and Julie, for example, in chapter 4, discussed the
need to treat the patient and not the protocol or the machine. In other
words, while the protocols may help workers avoid some very dangerous mistakes, Jake and Julie alluded to how the protocols and other
health technologies can seriously constrain workers' opportunities to
respond in ways that take into account the individuality and the family or social contexts of their patients. These consequences can be compounded with the instillation of managerial logics and a calculative
rationality (Clarke & Newman, 1997, p. 144; Cribb, 2008, p. 232) on and
off the streets of EMS; whereas, in the past, needs were determined by
both professional and bureaucratic judgments, today needs are being
organized by neoliberal rationalities that accentuate "margin over mis-
sion" (Weinberg, 2003, p. 17; Clarke & Newman, 1997) and therefore
decrease the quality of care patients receive (Rankin & Campbell, 2006;
Weinberg, 2003). Furthermore, there may be dangerous consequences;
Jake also discussed the need to "self-police" because of the increased
potential to do harm to their patients in light of the new protocols.

The possible changes to the professional mandate of paramedics
raise some interesting questions. Do these technologies and the discourses embedded within them represent a change in mandate that

may erode complex orientations that gear the work of paramedics towards the "what ifs"? Do these changes institutionalize discourses of good and bad patients, discourses that may be problematic for some types of patients? In other words, while it is likely that paramedics have always distinguished between "good" and "shit" calls, they are now being given the authority to act on this categorical understanding of calls, and by proxy, of patients, in ways that are now institutionally mandated. Will reform and restructuring practices inadvertently target specific groups of individuals, like patients who are more likely to appear in "shit" calls (e.g., intoxicated people, seniors, and people of lower socioeconomic status)? Will the institutionalization of "shit" calls displace the art of convincing patients to go to the hospital and instead instil a discourse of deserving and non-deserving patients? While these questions require more investigation, certainly the empirical evidence depicted throughout this book points to many of these consequences being realized on and off the streets for paramedics and for those with whom they interface.

One medical director I spoke with expressed another concern about how a "treat and refer" policy that would allow paramedics to divert certain patients away from the hospital might play out in practice:

> Once you get beyond some of the really simple clearly defined areas like hypoglycemia, it's much more difficult to actually validate the safety of an approach that involves leaving [patients] in the field. So, one of the ones that is under review right now is seizures, another one is asthma. The concern with asthma is that, you know, in most cases it's easy to diagnose, but occasionally there are people that present with wheezes that have other causes, so sometimes cardiac issues can cause wheezing, sometimes pulmonary embolism or blood clots in the lung can cause wheezes. So, problems that are not easily diagnosable or that may have, you know, confusing presentations really don't lend themselves to a treat and refer, treat and release approach, which is what, you know, we're hoping to expand upon. So, I personally have concerns if we're going to take that approach in terms of choosing certain patient cohorts that don't need to go to a hospital ... sometimes that's the most useful thing that we do from the emergency department perspective is rule out disease. That's something honestly that can't be done in the field and that a lot of these patients that have vague presentations are likely to be nothing. We can't tell you that it's nothing until we've had you in the emergency department for eight hours and done a million-dollar workup ... Paramedics are very good at

ruling in disease, but they're very poor at ruling out disease because disease is so complex.

The concerns expressed by this medical director are compounded by educational and training resources being "thin" throughout the province; resources that in the past were used for the city are now being spread throughout larger areas, therefore adding "way more players" without an increase in the resources. One field trainer explained that, since the takeover by the AHS, "the challenge is increased number of staff without a significant increase in resources to deal with the staff, and so basically how you get the training and education out to staff when you're continually being compromised as to how to do that with the limited resources that you have, so of course that was increased exponentially when we took over the province, right." Embedded in the talk of this field trainer is the concern that a thinning of education and training resources can impact the success of front-line workers. This is especially relevant in light of changing mandates and increased scopes of practice.

Reformation of Time

Linking these consequences is what appears to be a reformation of time in EMS, a reconceptualization that connects to Rothman's (1991) discussion of how "extra" beds in emergency departments were reconceptualized vis-à-vis discourses of efficiency. Rothman discusses how, before the entrance of third-party payers and players, "the idea of a 'surplus bed' did not carry the meaning that it now has" (p. 125); beds that were once viewed as hospital resources (p. 126) that were available when needed were reconceptualized to be viewed as a cost to be managed through quantitative technologies such as "length of stay" statistics (see Rankin and Campbell, 2006).

We saw in previous chapters that an important component of quality assurance is time, because "time is of the essence" in the medical and physiological sense; seconds can sometimes make the difference between life and death. However, we see that embedded within these reform and restructuring practices is a conceptualization of time that is at odds with the older version. Encroaching into the notion that "time is of the essence" are neoliberal notions of efficiency; efficiency is now central to the "essence" of time. In other words, time is, in part, being reconceptualized as "time is money" in order to garner cost efficiencies.

Facilitating the implementation of efficiency discourses into practice are technologies of knowledge and governance that produce standardized notions of work that interconnect with standardized notions of accountability. The technologies discussed in the previous chapters (e.g., REPAC, Emergency Medical Dispatch Protocols, ePCR, Lifepak), for example, create the potential to organize and monitor local happenings in relation to time more closely than ever before (DeVault, 2008). As previously mentioned, such technologies create very specific knowledge that, in the age of technological governance, is being funnelled into projects geared towards garnering efficiencies in health care.

While this conceptualization of time is not inevitably problematic, some paramedics I spoke with expressed concerns that it represented a downgrade in the quality of EMS. They specifically focused on concerns about the standards of response times in the city and how response times have become less important since AHS took over. One paramedic explained how "time" is not what it used to be:

> We've kind of thrown a lot of that out the window ... They wanted us to be at a life or death type of call within nine minutes, nine or ten minutes, 90 per cent or 80 per cent of the time; we're making that maybe 60. So they've kind of thrown it out. That was a big thing with the city. Chute times [the amount of time it takes paramedics to acknowledge to Dispatch that they are responding to a call] was everything ... Time wise there, it's something that's changed for management as well here now ... But yeah time's everything.

Alternatively, a stringent focus on time is not the solution either. Price (2006), for instance, discusses the consequence of eight-minute response times being introduced to paramedics in an attempt to improve patient outcomes for certain conditions. He found that such time measurements were problematic; paramedics in his study described the response times as "ludicrous," "an obsession," and "impossible" to meet. Furthermore, hidden consequences emerged. As one paramedic in his study explained, "We are now treating the clock and not the patient," resulting in an effect opposite to the original intent, not only putting patients at risk but also paramedics themselves (p. 128).

The point is that there are consequences for a system that is designed under the organizing principle of efficiency and cost-benefit ideologies and standardized notions of accountability; consequences that are likely magnified when it comes to life and death. While the technologies explored in previous chapters are institutionally thought and written about as leading to a more efficient use of resources, there are unaccounted costs in garnering efficiencies. Furthermore, while time is often essential to the work of paramedics and the quality of care patients receive, this focus on time must be complemented by other work processes of both patient and practitioner that move beyond simplistic assumptions of knowledge.

Broader Implications

By ethnographically exploring the work and workplace setting of paramedics, this book adds to the sociological literature on health, illness, and society. While the field of medical sociology is vast,[3] of particular relevance to this book is the sociological research on the work of health professionals, research that focuses primarily on the work and work settings of doctors and nurses. "Far less analysis," Schwartz (1994) notes, "has been carried out on relationships between patients and other kinds of health professionals" (p. 73). This is echoed more recently by Allen and colleagues (2016), who state, "sociological studies have for too long been preoccupied by the inner workings of medicine, and to a lesser extent nursing, with relatively little attention given to the work of others within healthcare" (p. 189). Furthermore, in the context of evidence-based medicine, Mykhalovskiy and colleagues (2008) point out that most research on "evidence-based health care management focuses on administrators, physicians or upper-level nursing staff" (p. 198). This book therefore provides important insights into the work of relatively new health care professionals and how their work interfaces with others in the health care system, as well as their workplace settings, from the standpoint of paramedics.

This book also contributes to research that focuses on how information and communication technologies (ICTs) (e.g., evidence-based medicine and dispatch protocols, REPAC, ePCR, etc.) organize work and knowledge relations in health care (see Lupton, 2014, for an overview). One of the main limitations of current research on ICTs is that the work of people disappears; what people are doing is objectified "above" local happenings, displacing the presence of people and their doings up to the conceptual "14th floor" (Smith, 2008, p. 418). Furthermore, ICTs are conceptualized in some of this research as a "third party to a conversation" (Ventres et al., 2006, p. 130) or as "non-human actors" (Lupton, 2014, p. 1348). However, as demonstrated throughout this book, ICTs do not simply act on their own. Rather, the technologies, and the discourses they carry, are activated by *people at work* (DeVault, 2008). This book explores not only how technologies are central to health care settings and to those on the front lines but also how technologies socially organize knowledge of that work in the age of technological governance.[4] In doing so, we can better understand how ICTs can be used as a "means of extending – socially, temporally, spatially – the technical rationality of the bureaucracy … connecting the *local, national and global in new ways*" (Hamilton, 2002, p. 104), as made visible in the diagrams in chapter 7.

Equally important, I have ethnographically looked beyond the promise of technological innovation and explored how technological "innovations" are part of social and political processes that have consequences, often hidden ones, for front-line workers and those they care for. Such implications suggest the need to be critical of taking a utopian or deterministic view of technologies (see MacKenzie & Wajcman, 2012) – a view that presents technologies as a simple solution to what are otherwise complex social problems[5] – and demonstrate a more "critical digital health studies" orientation that explores how technologies play out in practice (Lupton, 2014, p. 1347). Throughout part 2, I have problematized how technologies are often framed in health care discourse as a "solution" to societal problems and examined some of the "social, cultural, political and ethical dimensions of the digital health phenomenon" (p. 1347).

More broadly, this book contributes to the literature on the social organization of knowledge in health care that complements and critiques positivistic and quantitatively driven ways of knowing health care that predominate in contemporary reform and restructuring practices (Mykhalovskiy et al., 2008, p. 196). Similar to Diamond (1992) and Rankin and Campbell (2006), I provide an ethnographic look into how the work of health care workers has changed historically under the purview of health reform practices organized by ideologies of new public management and neoliberalism. By exploring and understanding the social organization of health care, the analysis undertaken in this book intersects with and organizes many of the substantive areas of interest to medical sociologists discussed above. The social organization of health care – the objectified forms of knowing based on ever-changing technologies of knowledge and governance that "organize and coordinate people's everyday lives" (Smith, 2005, p. 18) yet extend "outside the scope of the everyday world and are not discoverable within it" (Smith, 1987, p. 152) – organizes the medico-administrative complex (Mykhalovskiy, 2001) and the work of those who interface with it, including patients and practitioners.

Lastly, I would be remiss not to point out how this research blurs the lines between research on public health (traditionally thought of as preventing illness and promoting health) and EMS (traditionally thought of as services intended to treat illness). Much policy and practice in public health, for example, focuses on "risk" and "behaviourally oriented health promotion approaches" such as targeting "lifestyle" factors in order to promote health (Brassolotto, Raphael, & Baldeo, 2014, pp. 322, 323). This focus likely derives from the dominant discourses organizing health professionals, which are "usually biomedical, micro-level, individualized, and depoliticized" (p. 322; see also Raphael, 2011). This asociological orientation in public health is problematic, as Williams and Popay (1997) note:

> Some commentators have suggested that medical public health focused downstream to such an extent that it lost sight of what was going on up the river.[6] Moreover, public health research in general and clinical epidemiology in particular, increasingly excluded from its microscopic attention the voices of the people who in the words of Engels inhabited the "ruinous and filthy districts" within which the substances of bacteriology's scientific interest were festering. (p. 62)

As such, much research in the arena of public health is "flawed" (Coburn et al., 2003, p. 392); it is "context stripping" (Labonte et al., 2005, p. 8) of the intersectional social, political, and economic processes that structure health and illness in society (Brassolotto, Raphael & Baldeo, 2014). While this needs to be investigated further, I argue that we can learn much from the work of paramedics and other front-line workers that can add to research on public health. For instance, not only does studying the work of paramedics draw attention to the context in which individuals get hooked into the health care system, but also investigations of this type point to how paramedics engage with large-scale issues of health and inequality. The patients that paramedics treat and transport are not random; they are organized by social determinants of health (e.g., class, race, sex/gender, age, etc.). I suggest that the study of paramedics' work, and their workplace setting, can be seen as a canary in the mine, so to speak, of where society is failing its most vulnerable persons and hence can provide a lens to better understand the successes and failures of current public policies in Canada (and elsewhere) and systemic practices that organize the health status of individuals (see Low & Thèriault, 2008). Studying what paramedics do and their workplace settings allows a "deeper and more comprehensive understanding of people's experiences in their social, economic and political contexts" to emerge (Hills, 2000, p. I–4). Such a complex understanding of EMS may facilitate the "refocusing" of health policy and practice (and society) by pointing to where preventative and health promotional services and supports (generously conceived) could be directed (McKinlay, 1997).

Closing Remarks

Research of this type allows for "knowing health care" differently (Mykhalovskiy et al., 2008, p. 196). The empirical findings depicted throughout this book suggest a cause for concern in regard to how EMS is being reformed and restructured. With that said, this research offers no "silver bullet." My goal as a sociologist and institutional ethnographer is, in part, to offer an analysis that allows for a "talking back" in a similar fashion to Frank (1991) and Rankin and Campbell (2006); I hope that this research offers empirical evidence that responds to objectified forms of knowing by making visible complex work processes of paramedics and other front-line workers and explicating how their work processes are organized by powerful relations of coordination and control. In doing so, my goal is also to make visible how knowledge is socially organized in EMS and fill in some of the gaps that are part of the knowledge processes that demarcate "what counts." It is in this light that this research has a "democratizing potential" because it not only begins in the everyday work of paramedics but also "locates the effects of managerial initiatives in a broad political economy" (Mykhalovskiy et al., 2008, p. 201). I envision this conversation as an ongoing project of discovery that I hope front-line workers, like paramedics, and other individuals within and outside of the health care system will participate in.

In providing different types of empirical evidence – beyond a sole trust in numbers – my goal has been to diversify the type of knowledge that people who work in EMS settings can act upon. Since I am not a front-line health worker, the usefulness of this type of knowledge is an empirical question in and of itself. However, as Smith (2005) points out, findings from institutional ethnographic research like this can be used as an extension of what is already known about emergency medical services, and therefore provide health practitioners, administrators and managers, and policy makers alike with knowledge that will assist them in developing policies and practices that can facilitate the ongoing improvement of emergency medical services. As Marie Campbell (2010) explains: "Understanding how texts mediate the actions of health care personnel is crucial to analyzing health care problems ... That new 'solutions' also create new problems may not be self-evident" (p. 499; see also Weinberg, 2003, p. 14). The more the work of paramedics is made visible, the more responsive reforms can be to the actualities of front-line workers.

In offering a nuanced understanding of work processes and explicating the social organization that those work processes are embedded within, I have provided an alternative and more generous understanding of EMS work and the socially organized sites in which the work takes place. This exploration complements the stringent focus on quantitative ways of knowing (e.g., the chief complaint, event volume, and response time) in EMS and re-centres knowledge processes onto front-line workers. In doing so, I hope complementary understandings of "what counts" can emerge, whereby front-line workers and their work processes can become a part of, and thus balance out, other knowledge processes central to what gets counted. Ideally, this alternative narrative offers insights beyond the "hegemonic grip" (Diamond, 1992, p. 232) of simplistic and one-dimensional knowledge processes imbued with accounting logics that structure "what counts" in health care broadly and EMS specifically.

Notes

Chapter One

1 I use the term "paramedic" to refer to both Emergency Medical Technicians (EMTs) and Emergency Medical Technologist-Paramedics (EMT-Ps). I make distinctions when necessary.

2 http://www.sja.ca/English/About-Us/Pages/SJA-History-in-Canada.aspx, accessed April 2014.

3 http://www.qp.alberta.ca/documents/Regs/1993_048.pdf, accessed May 2016.

4 For an overview of the program, see http://www.sait.ca/programs-and-courses/full-time-studies/diplomas/emergency-medical-technology-paramedic-course-overview.php, accessed October 2015.

5 http://www.albertahealthservices.ca/728.asp, accessed June 2014.

6 http://www.albertahealthservices.ca/news/releases/2008/Page485.aspx, accessed January 2017.

7 http://www.health.alberta.ca/initiatives/health-action-plan-2008.html, accessed June 2014.

8 Nurok and Henckes (2009) researched pre-hospital workers in Paris and New York. In Paris, a pre-hospital unit is led by a physician and includes an "ambulance driver" and potentially other emergency personnel, like a nurse or a medical student. In New York, on the other hand, EMS units consist of paramedics or "First Aid" responders. According to Nurok and Henckes, the system in New York is designed for pre-hospital workers to "scoop and run" the patient from the scene to the hospital as rapidly as possible (p. 505). This is in contrast to the French system, sometimes referred to as "stay and play," where pre-hospital workers "provide on-scene stabilization of a patient to ensure transport to the hospital in the best condition possible" (p. 505).

9 See Bond et al. (2007), Canadian Association of Emergency Physicians Working Group (2002), Canadian Association of Emergency Physicians and National Emergency Nurses Affiliation (2003), Canadian Institute for Health Information (2005), Schull, Szalai, Schwartz, and Redelmeier, (2001), Skinner et al., (2008), Williams et al. (2001), Bird, Conrad, and Fremont (2000), Rothman (1991), and Wholey and Burns (2000).

10 For an overview of New Public Management's principles and logics, see Clarke and Newman (1997, p. 21) and Hunter (1996, pp. 801–2).

11 Closely connected to the concept of governance is Smith's concept of relations of ruling (see DeVault, 2008, p. 8).

12 I use the word "complex" throughout this book. Because of this, my use of this term needs to be clarified here. The word "complex" is a "blob" of sorts that holds very little, if any, meaning in and of itself (Smith, 2005). Nevertheless, I use this term for lack of a better word and attempt to fill it up with the work of paramedics as they interface with other people and different institutional sites of coordination and control. I therefore use the word "complex" relationally to the everyday doings of paramedics, which are contingent upon situational or contextual factors that add variance or difference to those doings. Suchman (2007) aptly points out the following in relation to this term: "In my view the complexity or simplicity of situations is a distinction that inheres not in situations but in our characterizations of them; that is, all situations are complex under some views and simple under others. Similarly, I cannot imagine what it could mean to deal with a situation in its 'full' complexity, because situations are not quantities of preexisting properties dealt with more and less fully. The point of the claim as reworded is just that *actions are structured in relation to specific circumstances and need to be understood in those terms*" (pp. 19–20, emphasis added).

13 I took a two-month "break" from riding along with crews (from May to June) following the birth of my twins.

14 This includes pairs where one crew member was the same as a previous ride-along but their partner for the shift was different.

15 I relied heavily on Emerson et al. (2011) to inform my approach to observations for two reasons: 1) They approach writing fieldnotes from a symbolic interactionist and ethnomethodological orientation (p. xvii), which aligns well with institutional ethnography because this orientation towards writing fieldnotes focuses on what people are actually doing, and 2) They emphasize writing fieldnotes as an anti-positivist process. With that said, while IE is rooted, in part, in ethnomethodology, as discussed above, it is also rooted in other commitments, which moves inquiry to

focus on how people's actual doings are socially organized. I refer to
Emerson et al. (2011) throughout this discussion, but as an institutional
ethnographer, I have other commitments as well that I oriented to
throughout my observations, data collection, and analysis.

Chapter Two

1 Paramedics also spoke of different training programs and how they
   vary in quality. For example, Julie explained to me after April passed her
   practicum that she "did not know how to set up some of the drugs when
   we asked her … She said, 'We never even got to open the drugs 'cause the
   [private school] was too cheap to open up drugs' … That leads to stupid
   students… The school that she [went] to has a reputation of doing that.
   They're private so you know, you watch the bucks."
2 I would also sometimes sit on the bench seat (next to the attending
   paramedic) or the seat opposite the attendant seat. Where I sat depended
   on the nature of the call, whether a student was riding along, and the
   preference of the paramedics I was riding with.
3 A flexible tube that can be inserted into the body.
4 I observed on a later call that the patient's chief complaint can organize
   not only the type of questions asked but also how a question is asked.
   For example, on a later call for a patient having "breathing problems,"
   instead of asking a combination of open-ended and yes/no questions, Jake
   primarily asked yes/no questions until the patient started to feel better.
5 I rarely saw paramedics flip through their protocol books. Through my
   observations, it became clear that they memorized the protocols and
   referred to the protocol book, or a phone application that had the protocol
   book downloaded on it, when necessary for clarification purposes.
6 Specific information must be entered into this computer, as indicated by
   the "yellow highlighted boxes" (Nurse Pam). Such information includes
   "first name, last name, location, so where you end up putting the patient,
   date and time … how they arrived …" (Nurse Pam). There is also a chief
   complaint box; Pam characterized this information as "just basically why
   the patient came in, and their symptoms, and what the medics did if it's a
   paramedic patient." She gave an example: "'Per EMS with complaints of
   chest pain since 0300 hours, no history of same, also short of breath and
   diaphoretic' and then I'll say something about the ECG, you know, 'There's
   changes in the ECG' for example. What else would I say? What the medics
   have given – 'Nitro x3 and ASA 160 given,' that kind of stuff, and then
   vital signs."

7 REDIS also provides the colour status of a hospital, which is supposed to indicate how busy the hospital is.

8 In relation to mechanisms of injury – "the mechanisms that are likely to cause injury" (Lerner et al., 2011, p. 2) or "how injuries happen" (Bahr & Krosshaug, 2005, p. 324) – and a motor vehicle collision, Julie might consider the following questions: "How did [the injury] happen? What kinds of speeds are we talking about? What kind of surface did they land on and how did they land on it?"

9 Similar to residents of long-term care facilities who sometimes appear "motionless," paramedics during their downtime, even if they are sleeping in between calls, are "actually moving and being moved through a social and political process" (Diamond, 1992, p. 74).

10 "Stretcher work" is considered an "occupational competency" of paramedics' work. For example, the Alberta Occupational Competency Profiles (AOCPs) identify the scope of practice for paramedics – what paramedics can and cannot do – depending on their designation (http://www.collegeofparamedics.org/practitioner-home/resources/faqs.aspx?faqID=2127, accessed February 2013). For each designation, paramedics are supposed to "practice safe lifting and moving techniques" and be able to "demonstrate proper body mechanics," which includes "body alignment, body balance, base of support, centre of gravity, coordinated body movement" with oneself and one's partner, and "communication with partner" (http://www.collegeofparamedics.org/wp-content/uploads/2016/04/aocp_emtp_full.pdf, accessed January 2017). This brief description provides snippets of understanding into how this work is actually accomplished on the ground and in practice.

Chapter Three

1 The Glasgow Coma Scale is used to assess the level of consciousness of patients. Fifteen is the highest score (meaning the patient is conscious and alert). One paramedic explained that a score of 15 means "he's speaking to us normally, and if I ask him to do something, he obeys commands. So he's a 15." This is in contrast to the score of three, which is lowest score possible, meaning the patient is unconscious and non-responsive. The same paramedic pointed to a chair and said, "This chair is a [three]."

2 I suspected that, in asking if he should give an additional 2.5 ml to the patient, Dan was deferring to Hanna's authority; even though both were EMT-Ps, Hanna had been an EMT-P for longer than Dan and was the senior crew member.

3 I put aside for now the potentially problematic assumptions and consequences of this prejudgment work because I am more interested here in how paramedics orient to certain patient characteristics, which further organizes and coordinates their work processes. With that said, there is much social scientific evidence that suggests such stereotypical patterns of beliefs can have an impact on how health practitioners treat their patients (see Chappell & Penning, 2009, p. 158). Clarke (2012) writes: "Considerable evidence demonstrates that the day-to-day practice of medicine is profoundly affected by social characteristics of both patients and doctors. First, with regard to patients, there is evidence that physicians tend to prefer younger patients and to hold negative images of elderly patients. Elderly patients tend to be seen as both sicker and less amenable to treatment than younger patients. The older patient ... 'represents the negative idea of the unco-operative, intractable, and generally troublesome patient' (Clark et al., 1991: 855) ... Physicians' attitudes and actions in regard to racialized characteristics reflect those of the wider socio-cultural context of which physicians are a part. For instance, several US-based studies have demonstrated that black patients tend to be referred to specialists less often, are treated more often by doctors-in-training, are more likely to be placed on a ward, and are admitted less frequently to hospital except when they are involuntarily hospitalized for mental health problems. Black patients also tend to receive less aggressive workups and interventions. Differences have also been documented in the way that physicians treat patients of different class backgrounds" (pp. 224–5).

4 While some might conceptualize what is described during this relief shift as an example of racism on the front lines of EMS, my goal here is to "ground" such concepts like "racism" in "social relations" (Smith, 2005, p. 57); rather than having such nominalizations like "racism," as traditionally conceptualized, stand in for or eclipse actual doings of people, my goal here is to explore "the ground of a concept in the actual ordering of what living people do" (Smith, 1990, p. 41). We see throughout these chapters how paramedics' work processes take shape through their work with different groups of individuals, for example, how paramedics are alert to certain things, how they prepare for a call and sometimes go in with certain assumptions, and how working with this "clientele" differs from working with other patients.

5 Another paramedic I spoke to voiced similar sentiments when he explained to me that once a patient is on the C-Spine board, "they need to get beds right away in the hospital."

6 According to Pam, "There's been full-on arguments up at triage about what's wrong with the patient and whether or not they're appropriate for the waiting room and then we have to get charge nurse and EMS supervisor involved, like it's happened."

7 We see in chapter 6 that there are some times when paramedic supervisors will enforce this policy more than others, like when Calgary "hits an alert."

8 Meg explained it as follows: "I have to say though at the [hospital I am currently at] I find it's very rare, and I'm not sure what the difference is between sites, but it's very rare that someone will really give me the wrong set of symptoms or the wrong story on a patient, and I'm not sure why; I don't know if they feel that they have to give the accurate thing because it's the trauma centre and there's so much going on there, I don't know. I do find there is a difference though and that I haven't had as many problems, although I've talked to other triage nurses and, you know after the medics have left and maybe they're waiting in the hall or they're doing whatever and you know I won't say much and then they'll say you know I really don't trust that medic."

9 http://www.albertahealthservices.ca/728.asp, accessed April 2014.

Chapter Four

1 I am reminded here of Edley and Wetherell's (1997) analysis of the work teenagers do in "jockeying for position" in the construction of their masculine identities.

2 This talk and the concerns raised by the paramedic who brought up this question exemplify a disjuncture of sorts that I wanted to learn more about: a disjuncture between the very non-standard work of paramedics and its complexity on the one hand, and on the other the institutional process of organizing, collecting, and standardizing front-line work (even though the protocols are supposed to be used in complex ways). This talk and part of this chapter allude to some of the problems that emerge when "knowing in text-mediated ways" (Campbell & Gregor, 2002, p. 36) is the primary way of being evaluated (the primary marker of evaluation) and accounting for work practices, whereas such text-mediated ways of knowing only represent a snippet of what actually happens (or the tip of the iceberg of actual work practices).

3 A field trainer explained that each protocol "actually says ... what an EMT could do, and what an EMR can do, what an EMT-P should do."

4 The Alberta College of Paramedics is the licensing body of paramedics in Alberta, which determines paramedics' scope of practice depending on

their designation (e.g., EMR, EMT, EMT-P). Jake explained that in Alberta, his full scope allows him to "basically administer about 98 different drugs and to do a whole lot more things than what my protocols allow me to do." We see in this talk that the protocols constrain him from working to his full scope of practice. He went on to say, "My protocols based on working for the city or for Alberta Health, they restrict some of those skills and I'm not allowed to use them."

5 Of course, convincing work did not apply to all situations; many patients were willing to be transported to hospital, but some were not. This description of work practices is geared towards the latter.

6 "With physician or law enforcement authorization," paramedics can "form" – take to the hospital against their will – "non-consenting patients" who pose a danger to themselves or others and/or are intoxicated and therefore "not considered competent." For example, patients can be "formed" under the Mental Health Act of Alberta if they meet three criteria: having a mental disorder, potentially causing harm to self or others, and refusing treatment (see AHS, 2010a).

Chapter Five

1 According to CIHI (2005), of the 12 per cent of patients arriving by ambulance to the ED in 2003/4, the majority (52 per cent) were individuals older than 85 years. Furthermore, patients with the "most severe health concerns" tended to be transported to the ED by EMS. With that said, adults between the ages of 16 and 64 accounted for the highest "absolute number of ED visits" at 61 per cent (p. vii). Lastly, a majority of visits to the ED (57 per cent) were for "less urgent conditions (for example, chronic back pain or minor allergic reactions) or non-urgent conditions (for example, sore throat, menses, or isolated diarrhea), based on the Canadian Triage and Acuity Scale (CTAS)" (p. vii).

2 I suspect that this is similar for doctors and nurses. For example, during one call, and after arriving in the hospital, a doctor came up to Jake and Julie while their patient was being triaged and asked, "Can I get a sneak peek? Anything exciting?" Jake and Julie tersely responded, "No." The doctor then walked away. See Becker (1993) for a discussion of good patients and "crocks."

Chapter Six

1 I identify individuals by the jobs they were performing when I was observing them or interviewing them. It is important to note that many

of the individuals I spoke with were cross-trained and therefore worked in different areas of the Centre. Many of the individuals I spoke with talked about the many different facets of the work that goes on in the Centre.

2 One call-taker manager explained that call-takers "are usually your more junior employees."

3 I enter pauses in this talk to give readers a sense of when the caller is speaking.

4 Some research is now suggesting that time is not always of the essence (see http://www.jems.com/article/ems-insider/great-ambulance-response-time-debate, accessed November 2015).

5 http://www.albertahealthservices.ca/ahs-nls-otm-2008-12.pdf, accessed November 2015.

6 REDIS provides data to the Canadian Institute for Health Information (CIHI)'s National Ambulatory Care Reporting System (NACRS). Such information is used by CIHI to "evaluate the management of ambulatory care services in Canadian health care facilities" (CIHI, 2011, p. 1).

7 See also Suchman's (2007) discussion on situated actions. For example, she writes, "humans dynamically coconstruct the mutual intelligibility of a conversation through an extraordinarily rich array of embodied interactional competencies, strongly situated in the circumstances at hand (the bounds and relevance of which are, in turn, being constituted through that same interaction). I accordingly adopted the strategy of taking the premise of interaction seriously and applying a similar kind of analysis to people's encounters with the machines to those being done in conversation analysis" (pp. 10–11). She also writes, "By situated actions I mean simply actions taken in the context of particular, concrete circumstances. In this sense one could argue that we all act like the Trukese, however much some of us may talk like Europeans. We must act like the Trukese because the circumstances of our actions are never fully anticipated and are continuously changing around us. As a consequence our actions, although systematic, are never planned in the strong sense that cognitive science would have it" (p. 26).

8 Svennevig (2012) explains that a caller who is a non-native speaker of the dominant language (in this example, an individual whose first language is not Norwegian) "normally requires additional efforts by the interlocutor in order to establish what has been said" (p. 1409).

9 http://www.albertahealthservices.ca/assets/about/ems/ahs-data-ems-event-calgary.pdf, accessed January, 2017.

10 We see in this chapter that people in the Dispatch Centre do anticipatory work.

Chapter Seven

1 http://www.albertahealthservices.ca/3165.asp, accessed January 2017.
2 This medical director explained that the protocols are an "indirect" or "prospective" form of oversight. A more direct form of oversight is known as "online" medical "consultation," whereby the paramedic in the street would phone a medical director. We saw this in chapter 4 when Julie consulted an emergency department physician about the patient who was passing in and out of consciousness.
3 See http://www.zoll.com/, accessed November 2015.
4 http://www.homeland1.com/homeland-security-products/ emergency-services-software/press-releases/344996-city-of-calgary-ems-partners-with-zoll-data-systems-to-improve-patient-care-with-electronic-patient-care-reporting/, accessed November 2015.
5 See http://www.medusamedical.com/, accessed November 2015.
6 http://www.medusamedical.com/SirenOverview/images/Siren-ePCR.pdf, accessed June 2013.
7 The quarterly reports, this individual explained, are primarily provided to upper-level administrators ("senior vice president level" and "up") at Alberta Health Services and Alberta Health and Wellness (now called Alberta Health).
8 The specialist explained that the performance measures "are sponsored by the EMS Chiefs of Canada." According to the EMS Chiefs of Canada, "developing comprehensive and meaningful measures of the care EMS provides means going well beyond merely tracking response times, which is only one aspect determining the quality of care EMS provides … Instead, EMS needs to develop appropriate clinical standards and patient outcome evaluators that will consistently capture every aspect of the quality of care that EMS provides. This will lead EMS to strive to provide better care, not just more efficient care" (Emergency Medical Services Chiefs of Canada, 2006, p. 17).
9 The business "data analytics" software that the performance management specialist is referring to is called "IBM Cognos 10," and is developed by IBM http://www.medusamedical.com, accessed June 2013.
10 http://www.ibm.com/developerworks/downloads/im/cognosbi/, accessed June 2013.
11 http://www.ibm.com/analytics/us/en/technology/cognos-software/, accessed January 2017.
12 http://www.redbooks.ibm.com/redbooks/pdfs/sg247912.pdf, accessed June 2013.

13 http://www.albertahealthservices.ca/6340.asp, accessed February 2014.
14 http://www.albertahealthservices.ca/org/ahs-org-accreditation-progress-report.pdf, accessed December 2013.
15 http://www.accreditation.ca/uploadedFiles/About_Us/Strategic_Plan/Accreditation%20Canada%20Strategic%20Plan%202010%20to%202013.pdf, p. 4, accessed December 2013.
16 http://www.accreditation.ca/accreditation-programs/qmentum/required-organizational-practices/, accessed December 2013.
17 http://www.accreditation.ca/accreditation-programs/qmentum/, accessed December 2013.
18 https://accreditation.ca/our-history, accessed January 2017.
19 Kelley and Hurst (2006) explain that it has "become commonplace for countries to formally assess and 'incentivize' the performance of their health care system" through the use of "comparable data" (p. 9).
20 http://www.cihi.ca/CIHI-ext-portal/internet/en/document/types+of+care/hospital+care/acute+care/dad_metadata, accessed December 2013.
21 http://www.cihi.ca/CIHI-ext-portal/pdf/internet/DAD_DATA_ELEMENTS_2013_2014_EN, accessed December 2013.
22 http://www.cihi.ca/CIHI-ext-portal/internet/en/document/types+of+care/hospital+care/emergency+care/NACRS_METADATA, accessed December 2013.
23 http://www.cihi.ca/CIHI-ext-portal/pdf/internet/NACRS_DATA_ELEMENTS_2013_14_EN, accessed December 2013.
24 https://www.cihi.ca/en/health-system-performance/performance-reporting/international/oecd-metadata, accessed December 2013.
25 Mykhalovskiy (2001) writes: "In recent decades in North America and Western Europe, population-based knowledges have been increasingly drawn upon in the work of managing and regulating health services. Among them, biostatistics, health services research, and clinical epidemiology rely heavily on statistical expertise in coming to know and intervene in the health and health care of populations. Their growing popularity in health-care reform initiatives is one mark of the increased significance that numerically-based forms of expertise have for contemporary governance in social life (Porter 1995; Rose 1991)" (p. 269).

Chapter Eight

1 The CHAPS program and this "treat and refer" policy connect to Rankin and Campbell's (2006) discussion of how information in health care

settings has been used to generate "standard 'classes' of patients [that] require standard efforts," thereby regularizing the work of front-line health care workers (p. 30).

2 http://www.health.alberta.ca/initiatives/5-year-plan-progress.html, accessed February 2016.

3 The field of medical sociology ranges from studies in illness experience, which focus on more micro-level understandings of illness experiences (Frank, 1991) to more macro examinations of medicine as a social institution (Freidson, 1970), to science and technology studies that focus on the social construction of science itself (Riessman, 1994, p. 192). For a comprehensive overview of medical sociology, see Bird, Conrad, and Fremont (2000), and Brown (1994).

4 It is important to note that some of the analytical goals of institutional ethnography connect to what some science and technology scholars are interested in exploring, including biosociality – how "new subjectivities [are made] based on medical-administrative categories rather than traditional social relations" (Hogle, 2008, p. 850).

5 This deterministic view "presents technology alone as being capable of shaping society's form. The social context of technical innovation and change is obscured, and the complexity of the interactions of social, scientific, technical, economic and cultural factors is oversimplified into a neat thesis about how a key technical innovation induces change in all of the other components of society" (Hamilton, 2002, p. 112).

6 The upstream/downstream metaphor can be explained as follows: "My friend, Irving Zola, relates the story of a physician trying to explain the dilemmas of the modern practice of medicine: 'You know,' he said, 'sometimes it feels like this. There I am standing by the shore of a swiftly flowing river and I hear the cry of a drowning man. So I jump into the river, put my arms around him, pull him to shore and apply artificial respiration. Just when he begins to breathe, there is another cry for help. So I jump into the river, reach him, pull him to shore, apply artificial respiration, and then just as he begins to breathe, another cry for help. So back in the river again, reaching, pulling, applying, breathing and then another yell. Again and again, without end, goes the sequence. You know, I am so busy jumping in, pulling them to shore, applying artificial respiration, that I have *no* time to see who the hell is upstream pushing them all in'" (McKinlay, 1997, pp. 519–20).

References

Accreditation Canada. (2009). *2009 Canadian health accreditation report: A focus on patient safety. Using Qmentum to enhance quality and strengthen patient safety.* Ottawa: Accreditation Canada.

Accreditation Canada. (2011). Canadian Health Accreditation Report: Quality Starts at the Top – The Pivotal Role of the Governing Body. Ottawa: Accreditation Canada. Retrieved from http://www.accreditation.ca/sites/default/files/char-2011-en.pdf

Alberta Health (AH). (2012). AAIMS batch data – Submission guidelines. Alberta Government. Retrieved from http://www.health.alberta.ca/documents/EHS-AAIMS-Batch-Data-Guidelines-V3-4.pdf. Accessed April 2014.

Alberta Health Services (AHS). (2010a). Emergency medical services provincial medical control protocols: Adult and Pediatric. Government of Alberta. Retrieved from http://www.emsccolorado.org/uploads/if-hp-ems-mcp.pdf

Alberta Health Services (AHS). (2010b). Becoming the best: Alberta's 5-year health action plan 2010–2015. Government of Alberta. Retrieved from http://www.health.alberta.ca/documents/Becoming-the-Best-2010.pdf

Alberta Health Services (AHS). (2011). Emergency medical services five year plan 2010–2015 – EMS: On the move. Retrieved from http://www.albertahealthservices.ca/assets/about/ems/ahs-ems-5-year-plan-2010.pdf. Accessed April 2014.

Alberta Health and Wellness (AHW). (2008a). Provincial service optimization review: Final review. Retrieved from http://www.health.alberta.ca/documents/Service-Optimization-Review-2008.pdf

Alberta Health and Wellness (AHW). (2008b). Vision 2020 – The future of health care in Alberta: Phase one. Retrieved from http://www.health.alberta.ca/documents/Vision-2020-Phase-1-2008.pdf. Accessed April 2014.

Allen, D., Braithwaite, J., Sandall, J., and Waring, J. (2016). Towards a sociology of healthcare safety and quality. *Sociology of Health & Illness, 38*(2), 181–97. http://dx.doi.org/10.1111/1467-9566.12390

Al-Shaqsi, S. (2010). Models of international emergency medical service (EMS) systems. *Oman Medical Journal, 25*(4), 320–3. http://dx.doi.org/10.5001/omj.2010.92

Armstrong, P., Armstrong, H., & Scott-Dixon, K. (2008). *Critical to care: The invisible women in health services.* Toronto: University of Toronto Press. http://dx.doi.org/10.3138/9781442687790

Bahr, R., & Krosshaug, T. (2005). Understanding injury mechanism: A key component of preventing injuries in sport. *British Journal of Sports Medicine, 39*, 324–9. http://dx.doi.org/10.1136/bjsm.2005.018341

Baker, R., MacIntosh-Murray, A., Porcellator, C., Dionne, L., Stelmacovich, K., & Born, K. (2008). *Calgary health region. High performing healthcare systems: Delivering quality by design.* Toronto: Longwoods Publishing.

Bakhtin, M. (1986). The problem of speech genres. In C. Emerson & M. Holoquist (Eds.), *Speech genres and other late essays* (pp. 60–102). Austin: University of Texas Press.

Barnett, J., Barnett, P., & Kearns, R. (1998). Declining professional dominance?: Trends in the proletarianisation of primary care in New Zealand. *Social Science & Medicine, 46*(2), 193–207. http://dx.doi.org/10.1016/S0277-9536(97)00150-0

Becker, H. (1993). How I learned what a crock was. *Journal of Contemporary Ethnography, 22*(1), 28–35. http://dx.doi.org/10.1177/089124193022001003

Bell, R. (2009). *The ambulance: A history.* Jefferson, NC: McFarland & Company.

Bergman, P. (2007). Emergency!: Send a TV show to rescue paramedic services! *University of Baltimore Law Review, 36*(2006–7), 347–76. http://dx.doi.org/10.1093/acprof:oso/9780199272235.003.0007

Bird, C., Conrad, P., & Fremont, A. (2000). Medical sociology at the millennium. In C. Bird, P. Conrad, & A. Fremont (Eds.), *Handbook of medical sociology* (5th ed., pp. 1–10). Upper Saddle River, NJ: Prentice Hall.

Bond, K., Ospina, M., Blitz, S., Afilalo, M., Campbell, S., Bullard, M., . . ., & Rowe, B. (2007). Frequency, determinants and impact of overcrowding in emergency departments in Canada: A national survey. *Healthcare Quarterly, 10*(4), 32–40. http://dx.doi.org/10.12927/hcq.2007.19312

Boyle, M., Williams, B., & Burgess, S. (2007). Contemporary simulation education for undergraduate paramedic students. *Emergency Medicine Journal, 24*(12), 854–7. http://dx.doi.org/10.1136/emj.2007.046318

Boyle, M., Williams, B., Cooper, J., Adams, B., & Alford, K. (2008). Ambulance clinical placements – A pilot study of students' experience. *BMC Medical Education, 8*(19). http://dx.doi.org/10.1186/1472-6920-8-19

Brassolotto, J., Raphael, D., & Baldeo, N. (2014). Epistemological barriers to addressing the social determinants of health among public health professionals in Ontario, Canada: A qualitative inquiry. *Critical Public Health, 24*(3), 321–36. http://dx.doi.org/10.1080/09581596.2013.820256

Brown, D. (2006). Working the system: Re-thinking the institutionally organized role of mothers and the reduction of "risk" in child protection work. *Social Problems, 53*(3), 352–70. http://dx.doi.org/10.1525/sp.2006.53.3.352.

Brown, P. (1994). Themes in medical sociology. In H. Schwartz (Ed.), *Dominant issues in medical sociology* (3rd ed., pp. 3–15). New York: McGraw-Hill.

Bureau of Labor Statistics. (2015). U.S. Department of Labor, *Occupational Outlook Handbook, 2016–17 Edition*, EMTs and Paramedics. Retrieved from https://www.bls.gov/ooh/healthcare/emts-and-paramedics.htm. Accessed January 12, 2017

Burns, L. (1994). The transformation of the American hospital: From community institutions toward business enterprise. In H. Schwartz (Ed.), *Dominant issues in medical sociology* (3rd ed., pp. 312–31). New York: McGraw-Hill.

Campbell, A. (2013). Work organization, care, and occupational health and Safety. In P. Armstrong & S. Braedley (Eds.), *Troubling care: Critical perspectives on research and practices* (pp. 89–100). Toronto: Canadian Scholars' Press.

Campbell, M. (2008). (Dis)continuity of care: Explicating the ruling relations of home support. In M. DeVault (Ed.), *People at work: Life, power, and social inclusion in the new economy* (pp. 266–88). New York: New York University Press.

Campbell, M. (2010). Institutional ethnography. In I. Bourgeault, R. DeVries, & R. Dingwall (Eds.), *Handbook on qualitative health research* (pp. 497–512). London: Sage Publications.

Campbell, M., & Gregor, F. (2002). *Mapping social relations: A primer in doing institutional ethnography*. Toronto: Garamond Press.

Campeau, A. (2008). Professionalism: Why paramedics require "theories-of-practice." *Journal of Emergency Primary Health Care, 6*(2), 1–7. Retrieved from http://pandora.nla.gov.au/pan/37708/20081028-0004/www.jephc.com/full_articled137.html?content_id=473

Canadian Association of Emergency Physicians & National Emergency Nurses Affiliation. (2003). Joint position statement on access to acute care in the setting of emergency department overcrowding. *NENA Outlook*, Spring, 15–19.

Canadian Association of Emergency Physicians Working Group. (2002). The future of emergency medicine in Canada: Submission from CAEP to the

Romanow Commission. Part 1. *Canadian Journal of Emergency Medicine*, 4(6), 359–68. Retrieved from http://www.cjem-online.ca/sites/cjem-online.ca/files/pg359(2).pdf

Canadian Institute for Health Information (CIHI). (2005). Understanding emergency department wait times: Who is using emergency departments and how long are they waiting? Retrieved from https://secure.cihi.ca/free_products/Wait_times_e.pdf. Accessed April 2014.

Canadian Institute for Health Information (CIHI). (2011). Data quality documentation for external users: National Ambulatory Care Reporting System, 2010–2011. Retrieved from http://www.cihi.ca/cihi-ext-portal/pdf/internet/nacrs_exec_summ_2010_2011_en. Accessed April 2014.

Chappell, N. McDonald, L., & Stones, M. (2008). *Aging in contemporary Canada* (2nd ed.). Toronto: Prentice Hall.

Chappell, N., & Penning, M. (2009). *Understanding health, health care, and health policy in Canada: Sociological perspectives.* Don Mills, ON: Oxford University Press.

Chung, C. (2001). The evolution of emergency medicine. *Hong Kong Journal of Emergency Medicine*, 8(2), 84–9.

Church, J., & Smith, N. (2006). Health reform and privatization in Alberta. *Canadian Public Administration*, 49(4), 486–505. http://dx.doi.org/10.1111/j.1754-7121.2006.tb01995

Clarke, J. (2012). *Health, illness, and medicine in Canada* (6th ed.). Don Mills, ON: Oxford University Press.

Clarke, J., & Newman, J. (1997). *The managerial state: Power, politics and ideology in the remaking of social welfare.* London: Sage Publications.

Clawson, J., Olola, C., Heward, A., Scott, G., & Patterson, B. (2007). Accuracy of emergency medical dispatchers' subjective ability to identify when higher dispatch levels are warranted over a Medical Priority Dispatch System automated protocol's recommended coding based on paramedic outcome data. *Emergency Medicine Journal*, 24(8), 560–3. http://dx.doi.org/10.1136/emj.2007.047928

Coburn, D., Denny, K., Mykhalovskiy, E., McDonough, P., Robertson, A., & Love, R. (2003). Population health in Canada: A brief critique. *American Journal of Public Health*, 93(3), 392–6. Retrieved from http://www.ncbi.nlm.nih.gov/pmc/articles/PMC1447750/

Cochrane, A. (2004). Modernisation, managerialism and the culture wars: Reshaping the local welfare state in England. *Local Government Studies*, 30(4), 481–96. http://dx.doi.org/10.1080/0300393042000318950

Corman, M. (2016). Street medicine – Assessment work strategies of paramedics on the front lines of emergency health services. *Journal of Contemporary Ethnography*, 1–24. http://dx.doi.org/10.1177/0891241615625462

Corman, M., & Melon, K. (2014). Managed professionals on the front line of emergency services. In D. Smith & A. Griffith (Eds.), *Governance on the front line* (pp. 148–76). Toronto: University of Toronto Press.

Cribb, A. (2008). Organizational reform and health-care goods: Concerns about marketization in the UK NHS. *Journal of Medicine and Philosophy, 33*(3), 221–40. http://dx.doi.org/10.1093/jmp/jhn008

Cromdal, J., Osvaldsson, K., & Persson-Thunqvist, D. (2008). Context that matters: Producing "thick-enough descriptions" in initial emergency reports. *Journal of Pragmatics, 40*(5), 927–59. http://dx.doi.org/10.1016/j.pragma.2007.09.006

Cromdal, J., Persson-Thunqvist, D., & Osvaldsson, K. (2012). "SOS 112 what has occurred?" Managing openings in children's emergency calls. *Discourse, Context & Media, 1,* 183–202. http://dx.doi.org/10.1016/j.dcm.2012.10.002

Daly, J. (2005). *Evidence-based medicine and the search for a science of clinical care.* Berkeley and London: University of California Press.

Daniel, Y. (2008). The "textualized" student: An institutional ethnography of a funding policy for students with special needs in Ontario. In M. DeVault (Ed.), *People at work: Life, power, and social inclusion in the new economy* (pp. 248–65). New York: New York University Press.

DeVault, M. (Ed.). (2008). *People at work: Life, power, and social inclusion in the new economy.* New York: New York University Press.

Diamond, T. (1992). *Making gray gold: Narratives of nursing home care.* Chicago: University of Chicago Press. http://dx.doi.org/10.7208/chicago/9780226144795.001.0001

Donnelly, E. (2012). Work-related stress and posttraumatic stress in emergency medical services. *Prehospital Emergency Care, 16*(1), 76–85. http://dx.doi.org/10.3109/10903127.2011.621044

Dopson, S., & Fitzgerald, L. (2005). Introduction. In S. Dopson & L. Fitzgerald (Eds.), *Knowledge to action? Evidence-based health care in context* (pp. 1–7). Oxford: Oxford University Press. http://dx.doi.org/10.1093/acprof:oso/9780199259014.001.0001

Ducey, A. (2009). *Never good enough: Health care workers and the false promise of job training.* Ithaca: Cornell University Press.

Edley, N., & Wetherell, M. (1997). Jockeying for position: The construction of masculine identities. *Discourse & Society, 8*(2), 203–17. http://dx.doi.org/10.1177/0957926597008002004

Emergency Medical Services Chiefs of Canada. (2006). The future of EMS in Canada: Defining the new road ahead. Retrieved from http://www.emscc.ca/docs/EMS-Strategy-Document.pdf

Emerson, R., Fretz, R., & Shaw, L. (2011). *Writing ethnographic fieldnotes*
(2nd ed.). Chicago, London: University of Chicago Press. http://dx.doi.org
/10.7208/chicago/9780226206868.001.0001

Farmer, P. (1996). On suffering and structural violence: A view from below. *Daedalus,*
125(1), 261–83. Retrieved from http://www.jstor.org/stable/20027362

Finn, J.C., Fatovich, D.M., Arendts, G., Mountain, D., Tohira, H., Williams, T.A., …
Jacobs, I.G. (2013). Evidence-based paramedic models of care to reduce
unnecessary emergency department attendance – feasibility and safety.
BMC Emergency Medicine, 13(13). http://dx.doi.org/10.1186/1471-227X-13-13

Frank, A. (1991). *At the will of the body: Reflections on illness.* Boston: Houghton
Mifflin Company.

Freidson, E. (1970). *Profession of medicine: A study of the sociology of applied*
knowledge. New York: Dodd, Mead & Company.

Giddens, A. (1997). *Sociology* (3rd ed.). London: Polity Press.

Goldman, B. (Host). (2008, April 25). Making room for new health care
players. Radio series episode of White Coat, Black Art. Toronto: CBC radio.

Hall, K. (2005). Science, globalization, and educational governance: The
political rationalities of the new managerialism. *Indiana Journal of Global*
Legal Studies, 12(1), 153–82. Retrieved from http://ijgls.indiana.edu
/category/volume-12-number-1/

Hamilton, P. (2002). From industrial to information society. In T. Jordan &
S. Piles (Eds.), *Social Change* (pp. 96–137). Oxford: Blackwell.

Health Quality Council of Alberta (HQCA). (2013). Review of Operations
of Ground Emergency Medical Services in Alberta: In Accordance with
Section 15(1) of the Health Quality Council of Alberta Act. Retrieved from
http://www.hqca.ca

Hills, M. (2000). Human science research in public health: The contribution
and assessment of a qualitative approach. *Canadian Journal of Public Health/*
Revue Canadienne de Santé Publique, 91(6), I-4–I-7. Retrieved from http://
www.jstor.org/stable/41994044

Hogle, L. (2008). Emerging medical technologies. In E. Hackett, O. Amserdamska,
M. Lynch, & J. Wajcman (Eds.), *The handbook of science and technology*
studies (3rd ed., pp. 841–73). Cambridge, MA: Massachusetts Institute of
Technology.

Hunter, D. (1996). The changing roles of health care personnel in health and
health care management. *Social Science & Medicine, 43*(5), 799–808. http://
dx.doi.org/10.1016/0277-9536(96)00125-6

Institute of Medicine (US). (2007). *Committee on the Future of Emergency Care*
in the United States Health System. Emergency medical services at the crossroads.
Washington, DC: National Academies Press.

Jackson, N., & Slade, B. (2008). "Hell on my face": The production of workplace il–literacy. In M. DeVault (Ed.), *People at work: Life, power, and social inclusion in the new economy* (pp. 25–39). New York: New York University Press.

Kelley, E., & Hurst, J. (2006)."Health Care Quality Indicators Project: Conceptual framework paper." OECD Health Working Papers, *No. 23*, OECD Publishing, Paris. http://dx.doi.org/10.1787/440134737301

Kilner, T. (2004a). Desirable attributes of the ambulance technician, paramedic, and clinical supervisor: Findings from a Delphi study. *Emergency Medicine Journal, 21*(3), 374–8. http://dx.doi.org/10.1136/emj.2003.008243

Kilner, T. (2004b). Educating the ambulance technician, paramedic, and clinical supervisor: Using factor analysis to inform the curriculum. *Emergency Medicine Journal, 21*(3), 379–85. http://dx.doi.org/10.1136/emj.2003.009605

Labonte, R., Polanyi, M., Muhajarine, N., McIntosh, T., & Williams, A. (2005). Beyond the divides: Towards critical population health research. *Critical Public Health, 15*(1), 5–17. http://dx.doi.org/10.1080/09581590500048192

Lerner, E.B., Shah, M.N., Cushman, J.T., Swor, R., Guse, C.E., Brasel, K., … Jurkovich, G.J. (2011). Does mechanism of injury predict trauma center need? *Prehospital Emergency Care, 15*(4), 518–25. http://doi.org/10.3109/10903127.2011.598617

Light, D. (2001). Cost containment and the backdraft of competition policies. *International Journal of Health Services, 31*(4), 681–708. Retrieved from http://www.ncbi.nlm.nih.gov/pubmed/11809005 http://dx.doi.org/10.2190/6BD1-3N67-MLGV-MY4T

Low, J., & Thèriault, L. (2008). Health promotion policy in Canada: Lessons forgotten, lessons still to learn. *Health Promotion International, 23*(2), 200–6. http://dx.doi.org/10.1093/heapro/dan002

Lupton, D. (2014). Critical perspectives on digital health technologies. *Sociology Compass, 8*(12), 1344–59. http://dx.doi.org/10.1111/soc4.12226

MacKenzie, D., & Wajcman, J. (2012). Introductory essay: The social shaping of technology. Retrieved from http://eprints.lse.ac.uk/28638/1/Introductory%20essay%20%28LSERO%29.pdf

Mannon, J. (1982). Participant observer roles in emergency medicine: Problems and prospects. Paper presented at the Annual Meeting of the North Central Sociological Association, Detroit, Michigan.

McCoy, L. (2006). Keeping the institutional in view: Working with interview accounts of everyday experience. In D. Smith (Ed.), *Institutional ethnography* (pp. 109–25). Lanham, MD: Rowman & Littlefield Publishers.

McCoy, L. (2008). Institutional ethnography and constructionism. In J. Holstein & J. Gubrium (Eds.), *Handbook of constructionist research* (pp. 701–14). New York: Guilford.

McCoy, L. (2009). Time, self and the medication day: A closer look at the everyday work of "adherence." *Sociology of Health & Illness, 31*(1), 128–46. http://dx.doi.org/10.1111/j.1467-9566.2008.01120.x

McKinlay, J.B. (1997). A case for refocusing upstream: The political economy of illness. In P. Conrad (Ed.), *The sociology of health and illness: Critical perspectives* (5th ed., pp. 519–33). New York: St Martin's Press.

McLeod, B., Zaver, F., Avery, C., Martin, D., Wang, D., Jessen, K., & Lang, E. (2010). Matching capacity to demand: A regional dashboard reduces ambulance avoidance and improves accessibility of receiving hospitals. *Academic Emergency Medicine, 17*(12), 1383–9. http://dx.doi.org/10.1111/j.1553-2712.2010.00928.x

Melon, K. (2012). Inside triage: The social organization of emergency nursing work. Master's thesis, University of Calgary. ISBN: 9780494879061.

Metz, D. (1981). *Running hot: Structure and stress in ambulance work.* Cambridge, MA: Abt Books.

Mykhalovskiy, E. (2001). Troubled hearts, care pathways and hospital restructuring: Exploring health services research as active knowledge. *Studies in Cultures, Organizations and Societies, 7*(2), 269–96. http://dx.doi.org/10.1080/10245280108523561

Mykhalovskiy, E., Armstrong, P., Armstrong, H., Bourgeault, I., Choiniere, J., Lexchin, J., . . ., & White, J. (2008). Qualitative research and the politics of knowledge in an age of evidence: Developing a research-based practice of immanent critique. *Social Science & Medicine, 67*(1), 195–203. http://dx.doi.org/10.1016/j.socscimed.2008.03.002

Mykhalovskiy, E., & Weir, L. (2004). The problem of evidence-based medicine: Directions for social science. *Social Science & Medicine, 59*(5), 1059–69. http://dx.doi.org/10.1016/j.socscimed.2003.12.002

National EMS Research Agenda. (2001). Retrieved from http://www.nhtsa.dot.gov/people/injury/ems/ems-agenda/EMSResearchAgenda.pdf. Accessed April 2014.

Nurok, M., & Henckes, N. (2009). Between professional values and the social valuation of patients: The fluctuating economy of pre-hospital emergency work. *Social Science & Medicine, 68*(3), 504–510. http://dx.doi.org/10.1016/j.socscimed.2008.11.001

Palmer, E. (1983a). "Trauma junkies" and street work: Occupational behavior of paramedics and emergency medical technicians. *Urban Life, 12*(2), 162–83. http://dx.doi.org/10.1177/0098303983012002003

Palmer, E. (1983b). A note about paramedics' strategies for dealing with death and dying. *Journal of Occupational Psychology, 56*(1), 83–6. http://dx.doi.org/10.1111/j.2044-8325.1983.tb00114.x.

Palmer, E. (1989). Paramedic performances. *Sociological Spectrum, 9*(2), 211–25. http://dx.doi.org/10.1080/02732173.1989.9981884.

Paramedics Association of Canada. (2011). National Occupational Competency Profile for Paramedics. Retrieved from http://www.paramedic.ca/uploaded/web/documents/2011-10-31-Approved-NOCP-English-Master.pdf.

Pence, E. (2001). Safety for battered women in a textually mediated legal system. *Studies in Cultures, Organizations and Societies, 7*(2), 199–229. http://dx.doi.org/10.1080/10245280108523558.

Price, L. (2006). Treating the clock and not the patient: Ambulance response times and risk. *Quality & Safety in Health Care, 15*(2), 127–30. http://dx.doi.org/10.1136/qshc.2005.015651.

Porter, T. (1995). *Trust in numbers: The pursuit of objectivity in science and public life*. Princeton: Princeton University Press.

Rankin, J., & Campbell, M. (2006). *Managing to nurse: Inside Canada's health care reform*. Toronto: University of Toronto Press.

Raphael, D. (2011) A discourse analysis of the social determinants of health. *Critical Public Health, 21*(2), 221–36. http://dx.doi.org/10.1080/09581596.2010.485606

Riessman, C. (1994). Women and medicalization: A new perspective. In H. Schwartz (Ed.), *Dominant issues in medical sociology* (3rd ed., pp. 190–211). New York: McGraw-Hill.

Rothman, D. (1991). *Strangers at the bedside: A history of how law and bioethics transformed medical decision making*. New York: Basic Books.

Roudsari, B., Nathens, A., Arreola-Risa, C., Cameron, P., Civil, I., Grigoriou, G., . . ., & Rivara, F. (2007). Emergency medical service (EMS) systems in developed and developing countries. *Injury, International Journal of the care of the Injured, 38*(9), 1001–13. http://dx.doi.org/10.1016/j.injury.2007.04.008.

Schull, M., Szalai, J.P., Schwartz, B., & Redelmeier, D. (2001). Emergency department overcrowding following systemic hospital restructuring: Trends at twenty hospitals over ten years. *Academic Emergency Medicine, 8*(11), 1037–43. http://dx.doi.org/10.1111/j.1553-2712.2001.tb01112.x.

Schwartz, H. (Ed.). (1994). *Dominant issues in medical sociology* (3rd ed.). New York: McGraw-Hill.

Shah, M. (2006). The formation of the emergency medical services system. *American Journal of Public Health, 96*(3), 414–23. http://dx.doi.org/10.2105/AJPH.2004.048793.

Skinner, B., Rovere, M., & Warrington, M. (2008). *The hidden costs of single payer health insurance: A comparison of the United States and Canada*. Vancouver: Fraser Institute.

Smith, D. (1987). *The everyday world as problematic*. Toronto: University of Toronto Press.

Smith, D. (1990). *The conceptual practices of power: A feminist sociology of knowledge*. Toronto: University of Toronto Press.

Smith, D. (2005). *Institutional ethnography: A sociology for people*. Toronto: AltaMira Press.

Smith, D. (2008). From the 14th floor to the sidewalk: Writing sociology at ground level. *Sociological Inquiry, 78*(3), 417–22. http://dx.doi.org/10.1111/j.1475-682X.2008.00248.x

Strauss, A., Fagerhaugh, S., Suczek, B., & Wiener, C. (1985). *Social organization of medical work*. Chicago: University of Chicago Press.

Suchman, L. (2007). *Human-machine reconfigurations: Plans and situated actions* (2nd ed.). Cambridge, New York: Cambridge University Press.

Suter, R. (2012). Emergency medicine in the United States: A systematic review. *World Journal of Emergency Medicine, 3*(1), 5–10. http://dx.doi.org/10.5847/wjem.j.issn.1920-8642.2012.01.001.

Svennevig, J. (2012). On being heard in emergency calls: The development of hostility in a fatal emergency call. *Journal of Pragmatics, 44*(11), 1393–412. http://dx.doi.org/10.1016/j.pragma.2012.06.001

Swanson, B. (2005). *Careers in health care* (5th ed.). Blacklick, OH: McGraw-Hill.

Timmermans, S., & Berg, M. (2003). *The gold standard: The challenges of evidence-based medicine and standardization in health care*. Philadelphia: Temple University Press.

Ventres, W., Kooienga, S., Vuckovic, N., Marlin, R., Nygren, P., & Stewart, V. (2006). Physicians, patients, and the electronic health record: An ethnographic analysis. *Annals of Family Medicine, 4*(2), 124–31. http://dx.doi.org/10.1370/afm.425.

Weinberg, D. (2003). *Code green: Money-driven hospitals and the dismantling of nursing*. Ithaca: Cornell University Press.

Whalen, M., & Zimmerman, D. (1990). Describing trouble: Practical epistemology in citizen calls to the police. *Language in Society, 19*(4), 465–92. Retrieved from http://www.jstor.org/stable/4168174 http://dx.doi.org/10.1017/S0047404500014779.

Wholey, D., & Burns, L. (2000). Tides of change: The evolution of managed care in the United States. In. C. Bird, P. Conrad, & A. Fremont (Eds.), *Handbook of medical sociology* (5th ed., pp. 217–37). Fremont, Upper Saddle River, NJ: Prentice Hall.

Williams, G., & Popay, J. (1997). Social science and public health: Issues of method, knowledge and power. *Critical Public Health, 7*(1–2), 61–72. http:// dx.doi.org/10.1080/09581599708409079.

Williams, P., Deber, R., Baranek, P., & Gildiner, A. (2001). From medicare to home care: Globalization, state retrenchment, and the profitization of Canada's health-care system. In P. Armstrong, H. Armstrong, & D. Coburn (Eds.), *Unhealthy times: The political economy of health and health care in Canada* (pp. 7–30). Toronto: Oxford University Press.

Wilson, D. (2007). Health promotion in Alberta: Many miles travelled, many miles to go. In M. O'Neil, A. Pederson, S. Dupere, & I. Rootman (Eds.), *Health promotion in Canada: Critical perspectives* (2nd ed). Toronto: Canadian Scholars' Press.

Zola, K. (1972). Medicine as an institution of social control. *Sociological Review, 20*(4), 487–504. http://dx.doi.org/10.1111/j.1467-954X.1972.tb00220.x.

Index

Milton Keynes UK
Ingram Content Group UK Ltd.
UKHW010939160524
442765UK00003BA/121